Feedlot Production Medicine

Editors

DANIEL U. THOMSON
BRAD J. WHITE

VETERINARY CLINICS
OF NORTH AMERICA:
FOOD ANIMAL PRACTICE

www.vetfood.theclinics.com

Consulting Editor
ROBERT A. SMITH

November 2015 • Volume 31 • Number 3

ELSEVIER

1600 John F. Kennedy Boulevard • Suite 1800 • Philadelphia, Pennsylvania, 19103-2899

http://www.vetfood.theclinics.com

VETERINARY CLINICS OF NORTH AMERICA: FOOD ANIMAL PRACTICE Volume 31, Number 3
November 2015 ISSN 0749-0720, ISBN-13: 978-0-323-41358-9

Editor: Patrick Manley
Developmental Editor: Meredith Clinton

Veterinary Clinics of North America: Food Animal Practice (ISSN 0749-0720) is published in March, July, and November by Elsevier Inc., 360 Park Avenue South, New York, NY 10010-1710. Subscription prices are $235.00 per year (domestic individuals), $326.00 per year (domestic institutions), $110.00 per year (domestic students/residents), $265.00 per year (Canadian individuals), $430.00 per year (Canadian institutions), $335.00 per year (international individuals), $430.00 per year (international institutions), and $165.00 per year (international and Canadian students/residents). To receive student/resident rate, orders must be accompanied by name of affiliated institution, date of term, and the signature of program/residency coordinator on institution letterhead. *Clinics* subscription prices. All prices are subject to change without notice. **POSTMASTER:** Send address changes to *Veterinary Clinics of North America: Food Animal Practice*, Elsevier Health Sciences Division, Subscription Customer Service, 3251 Riverport Lane, Maryland Heights, MO 63043. Customer Service (orders, claims, online, change of address): Elsevier Health Sciences Division, Subscription **Customer Service, 3251 Riverport Lane, Maryland Heights, MO 63043. Tel: 1-800-654-2452 (U.S. and Canada); 314-447-8871 (ouside U.S. and Canada). Fax: 314-447-8029. E-mail: journalscustomerservice-usa@elsevier.com (for print support); journalsonlinesupport-usa@elsevier.com (for online support).**

Reprints. For copies of 100 or more, of articles in this publication, please contact the Commercial Reprints Department, Elsevier Inc., 360 Park Avenue South, New York, NY 10010-1710. Tel.: 212-633-3874; Fax: 212-633-3820; E-mail: reprints@elsevier.com.

Veterinary Clinics of North America: Food Animal Practice is covered in *Current Contents/Agriculture, Biology and Environmental Sciences, MEDLINE/PubMed (Index Medicus),* and *Excerpta Medica.*

Contributors

CONSULTING EDITOR

ROBERT A. SMITH, DVM, MS
Diplomate, American Board of Veterinary Practitioners; Veterinary Research and Consulting Services, LLC, Greeley, Colorado

EDITORS

DANIEL U. THOMSON, DVM, PhD
Department of Diagnostic Medicine and Pathobiology, College of Veterinary Medicine, Kansas State University, Manhattan, Kansas

BRAD J. WHITE, DVM, MS
Associate Professor, Department of Clinical Sciences, College of Veterinary Medicine, Kansas State University, Manhattan, Kansas

AUTHORS

DAVID E. ANDERSON, DVM, MS
Diplomate, American College of Veterinary Surgeons; Professor and Head, Department of Large Animal Clinical Sciences, College of Veterinary Medicine, The University of Tennessee Institute of Agriculture, University of Tennessee, Knoxville, Tennessee

MICHAEL D. APLEY, DVM, PhD
Diplomate, American College of Veterinary Clinical Pharmacology; Frick Professor, Department of Clinical Sciences, College of Veterinary Medicine, Kansas State University, Manhattan, Kansas

J.T. FOX, DVM, MS, PhD
Veterinary Research and Consulting Services, LLC, Hays, Kansas

DEE GRIFFIN, DVM, MS
Beef Cattle Production Management Veterinarian, Great Plains Veterinary Educational Center; Nebraska Educational Center, University of Nebraska – Lincoln, Clay Center, Nebraska

LEEANN HYDER, DVM
Michigan State University, Southgate, Michigan

SAMUEL E. IVES, DVM, PhD
Associate Professor, Department of Agricultural Sciences, College of Agriculture, Science and Engineering, West Texas A&M University, Canyon, Texas

ROBERT L. LARSON, DVM, PhD, ACT, ACVPM-Epi, ACAN
Professor, Coleman Chair Food Animal Production Medicine, Department of Clinical Sciences, College of Veterinary Medicine, Kansas State University, Manhattan, Kansas

KIP LUKASIEWICZ, DVM
Production Animal Consultation LLC, Sandhills Cattle Consultants, Inc, Saint Paul, Nebraska

MATT D. MIESNER, DVM, MS
Diplomate, American College of Veterinary Internal Medicine; Associate Professor and Head, Agricultural Practices, Department of Clinical Sciences, College of Veterinary Medicine, Kansas State University, Manhattan, Kansas

TOM NOFFSINGER, DVM
Production Animal Consultation LLC, Benkelman, Nebraska

KARIN ORSEL, DVM, MSc, PhD
Diplomate, European College of Bovine Health Medicine; Department of Production Animal Health, Faculty of Veterinary Medicine, University of Calgary, Calgary, Alberta, Canada

DAVID G. RENTER, DVM, PhD
Professor and Director, Center for Outcomes Research and Education, Kansas State University, Manhattan, Kansas

JOHN T. RICHESON, PhD
Assistant Professor, Department of Agricultural Sciences, College of Agriculture, Science and Engineering, West Texas A&M University, Canyon, Texas

DAVID R. SMITH, DVM, PhD
Diplomate, American College of Veterinary Preventive Medicine (Epidemiology Specialty); Mikell and Mary Cheek Hall Davis Endowed Professor, Department of Pathobiology and Population Medicine, College of Veterinary Medicine, Mississippi State University, Mississippi State, Mississippi

MILES E. THEURER, DVM, PhD
Center for Outcomes Research and Education, Kansas State University, Manhattan, Kansas

EDOUARD TIMSIT, DVM, PhD
Diplomate, European College of Bovine Health Medicine; Department of Production Animal Health, Faculty of Veterinary Medicine, University of Calgary, Calgary, Alberta, Canada

BRAD J. WHITE, DVM, MS
Associate Professor, Department of Clinical Sciences, College of Veterinary Medicine, Kansas State University, Manhattan, Kansas

BARBARA WOLFGER, DVM, PhD
Department of Production Animal Health, Faculty of Veterinary Medicine, University of Calgary, Calgary, Alberta, Canada

AMELIA R. WOOLUMS, DVM, MVSc, PhD
Diplomate, American College of Veterinary Internal Medicine; Diplomate, American College of Veterinary Microbiologists; Department of Pathobiology and Population Medicine, College of Veterinary Medicine, Mississippi State University, Mississippi State, Mississippi

Contents

Preface: Feedlot Production Medicine   xi

Daniel U. Thomson and Brad J. White

Feedlot Processing and Arrival Cattle Management   323

Tom Noffsinger, Kip Lukasiewicz, and LeeAnn Hyder

 Videos on cattle management accompany this article

Acclimating newly arrived cattle in a feedlot setting can increase cattle confidence, reduce stress, improve immune function, and increase cattle well-being. Understanding cattle instincts and using low-stress handling techniques teaches cattle to trust their caregivers and work efficiently for them throughout the feeding period. These techniques should be applied with newly arrived cattle when they are unloaded, moved from the holding pen to the home pen, and handled inside the home pen. Low-stress handling during processing and a sound processing protocol based on cattle history and proper risk assessment can improve cattle health from the start of the feeding period.

Use of Antimicrobial Metaphylaxis for the Control of Bovine Respiratory Disease in High-Risk Cattle   341

Samuel E. Ives and John T. Richeson

Despite research and increased availability of antimicrobials, the prevalence and challenges associated with bovine respiratory disease (BRD) in stocker and feedlot operations remain. Preconditioned calves can better handle the transition from the origin ranch to the feedlot, yet there is incentive for buyers to purchase high-risk cattle at a reduced cost, and this is influenced by the proven efficacy and availability of antimicrobial metaphylaxis. The poor sensitivity of current BRD field diagnostic methods, typical pathogenesis of BRD, and labor issues are additional reasons to use metaphylaxis. Nevertheless, practitioners should consider comprehensive and novel approaches to judiciously guide decisions on metaphylactic use of antimicrobials.

A Systematic Review of Bovine Respiratory Disease Diagnosis Focused on Diagnostic Confirmation, Early Detection, and Prediction of Unfavorable Outcomes in Feedlot Cattle   351

Barbara Wolfger, Edouard Timsit, Brad J. White, and Karin Orsel

A large proportion of newly arrived feedlot cattle are affected with bovine respiratory disease (BRD). Economic losses could be reduced by accurate, early detection. This review evaluates the available literature regarding BRD confirmatory diagnostic tests, early detection methods, and modalities to estimate post-therapeutic prognosis or predict unfavorable or fatal outcomes. Scientific evidence promotes the use of haptoglobin to confirm BRD status. Feeding behavior, infrared thermography, and reticulorumen boluses are promising methods. Retrospective analyses of routinely collected treatment and cohort data can be used to identify cattle at risk of unfavorable outcome. Other methods have been reviewed but require further study.

Bovine Viral Diarrhea Virus–Associated Disease in Feedlot Cattle   367

Robert L. Larson

Bovine viral diarrhea virus (BVDv) is associated with bovine respiratory disease complex and other diseases of feedlot cattle. Although occasionally a primary pathogen, BVDv's impact on cattle health is through the immunosuppressive effects of the virus and its synergism with other pathogens. The simple presence, or absence, of BVDv does not result in consistent health outcomes because BVDv is only one of many risk factors that contribute to disease syndromes. Current interventions have limitations and the optimum strategy for their uses to limit the health, production, and economic costs associated with BVDv have to be carefully considered for optimum cost-effectiveness.

Feedlot Acute Interstitial Pneumonia   381

Amelia R. Woolums

Acute interstitial pneumonia (AIP) of feedlot cattle is a sporadically occurring respiratory condition that is often fatal. Affected cattle have a sudden onset of labored breathing. There is no confirmed effective treatment of feedlot AIP; however, administration of antibiotics effective against common bacterial respiratory pathogens and nonsteroidal anti-inflammatory drugs, especially aspirin, has been recommended. Protective strategies are not well defined, but efforts to limit dust exposure and heat stress to ensure consistent formulation, mixing, and delivery of feed; and to identify and treat infectious respiratory disease in a timely manner, may decrease rates of feedlot AIP.

Investigating Outbreaks of Disease or Impaired Productivity in Feedlot Cattle   391

David R. Smith

Most cattle move through cattle feeding and finishing systems without health problems or impairment of productivity, but some cattle do become ill or unproductive. When cattle get sick, understanding what has gone wrong and how to remedy the situation is important. An orderly, systematic approach to investigating disease outbreaks is more likely to lead to a solution. The solution may come from identifying and modifying human decisions or behaviors that may be far removed in time or place from the immediate problem. Veterinarians can help cattle feeders recognize and correct the system dynamics factors affecting cattle health and performance.

Surgical Management of Common Disorders of Feedlot Calves   407

Matt D. Miesner and David E. Anderson

Procedures to improve animal and handler safety, shape production parameters, and directly address the prosperity of individuals in need of assistance are performed routinely. Techniques to accomplish these tasks have been described in many venues. Painful procedures are expected in feedlot practice. Assessing and managing pain and welfare for these procedures has strengthened significantly over the past decade to address increased public concerns and also to support the desires of the operators/managers to progress. Methods to perform common procedures are described, including evidence and techniques for managing the pain and distress while performing them.

Surgical Management of Orthopedic and Musculoskeletal Diseases of Feedlot Calves

425

David E. Anderson and Matt D. Miesner

Injuries, infections, and disorders of the musculoskeletal system are common in feedlot calves. These conditions often are amenable to surgical treatment with return of the calf to productivity. Weight gain and carcass quality are expected to be significantly adversely affected by pain and debilitation. The goal of surgical management of disorders of the joints, muscles, and feet should be resolution of the inciting cause, mitigation of pain, and restoration of form and function. If these are achieved, calves should return to acceptable, if not normal, feed intake, rate of gain, and carcass quality.

Treatment of Calves with Bovine Respiratory Disease: Duration of Therapy and Posttreatment Intervals

441

Michael D. Apley

When treating bovine respiratory disease, it is important to consider the decision to initiate treatment, the treatment regimen used, and whether to continue treatment. It is necessary to define the duration of drug exposure and when a success/failure decision will be made. No data are available to define the optimal duration of antimicrobial exposure. A pattern seen in human pneumonia studies is that shorter durations of therapy were equivalent with longer durations. Some studies suggest defining success or failure based on pharmacokinetics and pharmacodynamics may lead to earlier than optimal intervention. Optimal intervals are best defined by randomized clinical trials.

Management of Feedyard Hospitals

455

J.T. Fox

There are many considerations when managing feedyard hospitals. The type of hospital system must fit the facility design, the type of cattle fed at the feedyard, the crew that is employed by the feedyard, and the protocol established by the veterinarian. Ensuring the animals are well-cared for and have their basic needs met should be the priority of the feedyard personnel, and the veterinarian maintaining the veterinarian-client-patient relationship with the feedyard.

Feedlot Euthanasia and Necropsy

465

Dee Griffin

Timely euthanasia of feeder cattle can minimize suffering of cattle that have little hope of recovery or pain abatement. Euthanasia techniques are described, including primary and secondary steps to ensure humane death. Considerations are discussed to ensure rendered product from euthanized cattle will be safe. A necropsy technique that is time efficient and thorough is outlined. An important aspect is minimizing the number of detached body organs, thereby making it easier to remove the necropsied animal. A necropsy data collection system that uses check-boxes to record findings is discussed. A link to a database that can be downloaded is included.

Optimizing Feedlot Diagnostic Testing Strategies Using Test Characteristics, Disease Prevalence, and Relative Costs of Misdiagnosis   483

Miles E. Theurer, Brad J. White, and David G. Renter

Diagnostic tests are commonly used by feedlot practitioners and range from clinical observations to more advanced physiologic testing. Diagnostic sensitivity and specificity, estimated prevalence in the population, and the costs of misdiagnoses need to be considered when selecting a diagnostic test strategy and interpreting results. This article describes methods for evaluating diagnostic strategies using economic outcomes to evaluate the most appropriate strategy for the expected situation. The diagnostic sensitivity and specificity, and expected prevalence influence the likelihood of misdiagnosis in a given population, and the estimated direct economic impact can be used to quantify differences among diagnostic strategies.

Using Feedlot Operational Data to Make Valid Conclusions for Improving Health Management   495

Miles E. Theurer, David G. Renter, and Brad J. White

Feedlot operational data can be useful for monitoring cattle health and performance outcomes and evaluating associations between these outcomes and potentially important cattle population or management factors. Operational data are inherently relevant to clients; however, there are potential limitations that need to be considered to make appropriate conclusions. Assessing data quality, potential for bias, data distributions, and multiple health outcomes can provide a more thorough understanding of feedlot cattle health and factors that may affect health management systems. Accurate and useful information is derived only when the advantages and limitations of the data and the analysis process are fully understood.

Index   509

VETERINARY CLINICS OF NORTH AMERICA: FOOD ANIMAL PRACTICE

FORTHCOMING ISSUES

March 2016
Update on Ruminant Ultrasound
Sébastien Buczinski, *Editor*

July 2016
Bovine Theriogenology
Robert L. Larson, *Editor*

November 2016
Bovine Surgery
David Anderson and Andrew Niehaus, *Editors*

RECENT ISSUES

July 2015
Feedlot Processing and Arrival Cattle Management
Brad J. White and Daniel U. Thomson, *Editors*

March 2015
Bovine Clinical Pharmacology
Michael D. Apley, *Editor*

November 2014
Dairy Nutrition
Robert J. Van Saun, *Editor*

ISSUE OF RELATED INTEREST

Veterinary Clinics of North America: Small Animal Practice
September 2015 (Vol. 45, Issue 5)
Perioperative Care
Lori S. Waddell, *Editor*

THE CLINICS ARE NOW AVAILABLE ONLINE!
Access your subscription at:
www.theclinics.com

Preface

Feedlot Production Medicine

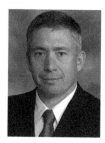 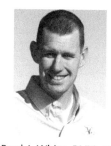

Daniel U. Thomson, DVM, PhD   Brad J. White, DVM, MS
Editors

Feedlot production medicine is a balance of animal husbandry, veterinary medicine, and economics. Veterinarians continue to focus on individual animal medicine while incorporating the influence of the cattle population on current or future issues. Beef cattle health and well-being in feedlot operations is dependent on processing crews, pen riders, and feedlot doctors working with other crews on the yard to provide consistent cattle monitoring and care.

This publication has brought feedlot experts across the United States and Canada together to discuss feedlot production medicine. Processing protocols, cattle handling, and the use of antibiotics to control and prevent bovine respiratory disease are imperative to getting cattle off to a good healthy start in the feedlot. Once cattle are moved out into the feeding pens, day-to-day management of monitoring cattle health and identifying sick or injured cattle is important for treatment success and economic performance. Biosecurity and diagnostic evaluations are important to disease investigation in understanding bovine viral diarrhea, atypical interstitial pneumonia, bovine respiratory disease, and other issues that impact cattle health and performance. A large focus of this publication discusses the importance of proper diagnostics, clinical definitions, and treatment protocols teamed with animal husbandry to manage cattle health through the feedlot production phase.

Many people debate the relevance of individual animal medicine versus population medicine when it comes to feedlot cattle health. Production medicine requires knowledge of both individual (clinical) and population (diagnostic) medicine combined with an understanding of the different production systems and management styles to provide the best health program for beef cattle. The issues surrounding feedlot cattle production can be influenced by the cattle procured, the people employed at the operation, and the environmental conditions. Balancing these variables with cattle disease and injury is an important factor in the decision-making for a feedlot veterinarian. Making the proper diagnosis at necropsy, identifying the proper animal in the feeding pen for treatment, administering the proper treatment based on clinical presentation,

Vet Clin Food Anim 31 (2015) xi–xii
http://dx.doi.org/10.1016/j.cvfa.2015.08.001
0749-0720/15/$ – see front matter © 2015 Published by Elsevier Inc.

and providing supportive care for the sick and injured animals are all part of a production medicine system. Feedlot managers, veterinarians, and the feedlot staff must communicate on all parts to make the best animal health, production, and economic decisions.

Beef cattle health is a cornerstone to feedlot cattle production systems. Animal husbandry, diagnostic medicine, clinical medicine, economics, and communication between feedlot personnel are very important pieces to a feedlot production medicine program. Many people work hard on a day-to-day basis to provide care and well-being for the cattle in the feedlots in North America. We hope this issue of the *Veterinary Clinics of North America: Food Animal Practice* serves the beef cattle veterinarians, ranchers, and feedlot operators in their business.

Daniel U. Thomson, DVM, PhD
Department of Diagnostic Medicine
and Pathobiology
College of Veterinary Medicine
Kansas State University
1800 Denison Avenue
Manhattan, KS 66506, USA

Brad J. White, DVM, MS
Department of Clinical Sciences
College of Veterinary Medicine
Kansas State University
1800 Denison Avenue
Manhattan, KS 66506, USA

E-mail addresses:
dthomson@vet.k-state.edu (D.U. Thomson)
bwhite@vet.k-state.edu (B.J. White)

Feedlot Processing and Arrival Cattle Management

Tom Noffsinger, DVM[a],*, Kip Lukasiewicz, DVM[b], LeeAnn Hyder, DVM[c]

KEYWORDS

- Acclimation • Processing • Stress • Handling • Induction

KEY POINTS

- Proper acclimation through low-stress cattle handling encourages timely rehydration, nourishment, and rest and improves immune function and cattle confidence.
- Acclimation involves proper handling when unloading cattle, emptying holding pens, moving cattle to the home pen, and handling cattle inside the home pen.
- Processing procedures depend on cattle history and risk and may include identification, parasite control, vaccination, hormone implantation, pregnancy management, castration, and treatment.

Videos on cattle management accompany this article at http://www.vetfood.theclinics.com/

INTRODUCTION

Arrival cattle management at feedlots is an exciting opportunity to decrease stress, shape cattle behavior, facilitate arrival processing product response, and initiate the training of cattle to work for caregivers. Producers have a simple choice. New cattle can be put in a pen and ignored, or caregivers can seize the exciting opportunities associated with new arrivals. Specific activities to be undertaken depend on cattle origin, history, arrival risk categories, and arrival behavior. However, understanding a process known as acclimation is key for optimal arrival management of cattle.

THE PURPOSE OF ACCLIMATION

Acclimation is the process and result of proper caregiver-cattle interaction that allows cattle to accept their new home environment. Caregivers demonstrate to cattle that

The authors have nothing to disclose.
[a] Production Animal Consultation LLC, 34122 Highway 34, PO Box 128, Benkelman, NE 69021, USA; [b] Production Animal Consultation LLC, Sandhills Cattle Consultants, Inc, 1306 Bruce Street, Saint Paul, NE 68873, USA; [c] Michigan State University, 15400 Brest Street, Southgate, MI 48195, USA
* Corresponding author.
E-mail address: dvm.drtom@gmail.com

they understand cattle instincts and sensory systems and can effectively communicate with the new arrivals. The performance and health goals of acclimation efforts with newly arrived cattle in feedlots are to provide rehydration, nourishment, and rest and to improve immune function.

Water is the most important nutrient for any animal. Yet often times, cattle have been without food and water for 24 to 48 hours before arrival at a feedlot, leading to dehydration. Richeson and colleagues[1] evaluated the hematocrit of cattle arriving at a feedlot and found the range to be 23.5% to 46.9%, with a mean hematocrit of $36.9 \pm 3.7\%$. The tendency for cattle to exhibit an elevated hematocrit at arrival is consistent with dehydration. Caregivers must make rehydration a priority for new arrivals because cattle depend on water to carry out basic metabolic functions. Dehydrated cattle are also reluctant to eat. Inadequate consumption of safe water can negatively affect feed intake, health, and production.[2–4] Brew and colleagues[5] found increased water intake was correlated with increased average daily gain (ADG) and increased feed intake in growing beef cattle. Preston[6] concluded that providing water to calves shortly after arrival increases feed intake to appropriate levels (greater than 1% of body weight) more quickly than providing feed alone.

The requirements for timely rehydration include access to fresh clean water, complete confidence in the new environment, and confidence in the new caregivers. Cattle that are not confident in their new space are reluctant to be confident in the water supply. Caregivers need to be aware that proper caregiver-cattle interactions can have a positive impact on pen distribution and willingness to aggressively drink. There is huge potential within the industry to install tank flowmeters that would allow the monitoring of daily water intake. Average water intake can vary from 25 to 35 L/head/d.[5] Systems such as GrowSafe (GrowSafe Systems Ltd, Airdrie, AB, Canada) enable producers to measure individual animals' food and water intake, even when they are housed in a group pen, through use of radiofrequency identification technology.[5] Efforts to document water intake levels as a predictor of future health and performance could help identify priority pens and validate caregiver acclimation progress.

In addition to being without water, cattle typically do not have access to feed during transport to the feedlot. The combination of transport and lack of food and water leads to decreased body weight beyond that associated with lack of food and water alone. Falkenberg and colleagues[7] found relocated cattle that had food and water withheld up to 12 hours had up to a 6% decrease in body weight compared with cattle that were starved but were not relocated that had a 2% decrease in body weight. Historically, intake expectations have been accepted less than 1% of body weight for multiple days after arrival to a feedlot, especially in high-risk, stressed arrivals. Yet dry matter intake levels to meet daily requirements are usually between 1.1% and 1.7% of body weight, varying with ration formulation. Caregivers and nutritionists should jointly elevate expectations for calves to have proper intakes from day 1. Total intake levels expressed as an average for the pen are important, but more important is the observation that all herd members are participating equally. Trained caregivers can facilitate uniform bunk activity via pen acclimation procedures within herds of new arrivals. Starter diets should be formulated to provide appropriate levels of protein, energy, trace minerals, and vitamins from commodities friendly to the ruminant digestive system. Donovan and colleagues[8] found that "lymphocytes from calves that were ketotic or acidotic exhibited a generally decreased responsiveness to superantigen stimulus." Acidotic and ketotic states can result from an improperly formulated diet with energy excess and improper intakes that lead to energy deficits, respectively. Handler promotion of proper intake can prevent these detrimental energy imbalances.

Transport prevents lying down and resting behavior in cattle, which can lead to increased stress levels and an increased risk for lameness. Although normal resting behavior has not been well documented, Calderon and Cook[9] found that, in dairy cattle, it is "influenced by calving month, temperature humidity index, body condition, parity, and lameness." Other studies have shown a variation in average lying time in dairy cattle between 9.6 and 13 h/d.[9,10] Several studies have shown when dairy cattle are deprived of lying for long or repeated periods they can have a decrease in growth hormone concentrations and an increase in levels of adrenocorticotropic hormone (ACTH),[10] a measure of cortisol that is increased in stressed animals. Cooper and colleagues[10] showed that after deprivation of time to lie down, dairy cattle spent more time standing without ruminating. Another study showed very low lying times have been associated with higher incidences of lameness in dairy cattle.[11] It is evident from these studies that deprivation of rest has harmful effects on the health and well-being of cattle. Caregivers should recognize that the amount of rest cattle have received is affected by the distance shipped. It is the responsibility of caregivers to encourage new arrivals to rest through caregiver-cattle interaction, bedding, and pen surface management.

Relocating to a new home is a major stressor in the life of an animal, and it has been well documented that such stress causes a decrease in immune function. Griffin and colleagues[12] note that the nasal passages of stressed animals often have higher densities of bacteria that cause bovine respiratory disease (BRD).[13,14] In addition, the temporary increase in plasma cortisol levels caused by transportation stress may be associated with increased risk for BRD.[12,15] A decrease in the circulating levels of acute phase proteins haptoglobin and fibrinogen found by Buckham Sporer and colleagues[16] provides further evidence of immunosuppression in transported cattle. Buckham Sporer and colleagues[17] evaluated the effects of elevated cortisol levels on neutrophil expression genes Fas, MMP-9, BPI, and L-selectin. Fas, a proapoptotic gene, was downregulated in response to elevated cortisol levels during transport, whereas MMP-9 (involved in tissue remodeling) and BPI (responsible for bacterial killing) were upregulated. L-Selectin is responsible for the vascular margination of neutrophils, and levels of L-selectin were decreased during transport, leading to an increase in the number of circulating neutrophils. Neutrophils that express L-selectin have preferential migration into the respiratory tract.[17] According to Buckham Sporer and colleagues,[17] "the elevated expression of MMP-9…may imply an increased potential for neutrophils to cause excessive inflammatory damage in infected lungs during transportation stress, which may be augmented further by the cells' reprogramming for longer lifespan (depressed Fas expression)." Increased migration of neutrophils with increased bactericidal activity into the respiratory system can result in the "'neutrophil paradox'…whereby these normally beneficial leukocytes can also contribute to the pathogenesis of infectious diseases if their proinflammatory activities are not properly regulated."[17] Thus, stressed cattle entering a feedlot are at higher risk of BRD and other diseases. Acclimation of cattle to their new environment can reduce anxiety and help to relieve some of the stress they experience, improving immune function and health.

HOW TO ACCLIMATE CATTLE

The primary focus of acclimation is stress reduction. The signs of stress are many, and stressed animals exhibit a mixture of these signs. Stressed cattle are often wary of their surroundings and their new caregiver. They tend to be herd bound and congregate in a chosen corner of their new pen. These animals keep whatever and whomever they view as a threat in their line of vision. Stressed cattle have spacious flight zones and are reluctant to pass by or engage with a handler. These animals are reluctant to travel in straight lines and exhibit aimless circling. Stressed cattle may or may not vocalize or exhibit decreased abdominal fill. One of the main negative effects of stressed animals is that they hide subtle signs of injury and disease. Cattle are a prey species and do not wish to be identified by what they consider a threat. Until cattle trust their caregiver, the caregiver is viewed as a threat and cattle do not present disease symptoms honestly.

Cattle in the process of relocation search for guidance and instruction. Positive first impressions are an efficient way to improve cattle confidence and create proper animal behavior. Greeting cattle as they file off a truck or trailer or into their new pen is an appropriate first step. Cattle crave to easily visualize their source of guidance and their destination simultaneously (Video 1). By positioning themselves to accommodate this instinct, handlers can start the process of convincing cattle they can pass by without incurring harm. Handler posture can also be used to convince cattle to trust the handler and to accept increasing degrees of pressure. Sensitive cattle refuse to pass by a handler with frontal focus; instead, handlers should turn their shoulder, side, or back toward the cattle. A relaxed posture is more encouraging than a confrontational, rigid, fixed posture with a puffed-up chest and broad shoulders. Handlers should encourage cattle to pass by through the application of the least amount of pressure that is effective in initiating and maintaining movement. Owing to poor depth perception, cattle are suspicious of handlers that stand still. Gentle swaying movements by handlers convince cattle that handlers understand their lack of depth perception and are willing to be clearly visible.

Once unloading is complete, it is time to send cattle to their new home pen. Proper emptying of the holding pen is the first step in this process. As handlers approach the holding pen, they should respond to the first signs of cattle acknowledgment by halting or changing angles. The most sensitive cattle in the holding area acknowledge handler presence by either raising their heads or moving away. The goal is for handlers to create orderly cattle flow out of the holding pen by working near the gate. The handler should enter the pen and move along the side of the pen that allows cattle to see the handler and their destination simultaneously (**Fig. 1**). As soon as cattle initiate motion, the handler should release pressure. Cattle choose to turn around

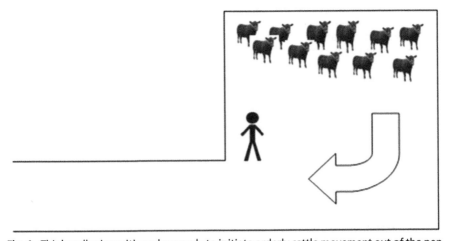

Fig. 1. This handler is positioned properly to initiate orderly cattle movement out of the pen.

the handler as they enter the alley (Video 2); this prevents them from rushing out of the pen, losing their footing, and striking their shoulders or hips as they exit.

Cattle should move into their new home pen voluntarily. If possible, allow cattle to go past their designated gate and volunteer to stop at a check gate or at the end of a drover's alley. Cattle instinctively return in the direction they came from; this creates voluntary motion and provides another opportunity to show cattle they can safely pass by a handler into their new home. After the cattle have volunteered to stop at the check gate or end of the drover's alley, the caregiver can then ask the cattle to move into their new home pen (Video 3). The caregiver should interact with the animals at the front of the group. Gentle pressure within the flight zone should be applied to ask the animals at the front to move past the caregiver. Once the first animal begins moving forward, the caregiver should move with that animal to relieve pressure from the remainder of the group. This action allows the caregiver to guide the front of the group while the remaining cattle follow. Because new cattle tend to have a large flight zone, being in the alley with them can place excessive pressure on these animals. Cattle that are under too much pressure turn into the check gate, press against their herd mates, and avoid eye contact with the handler. In these cases, the handler should move out of the alley and work with the cattle from a neighboring pen (**Fig. 2**). Gently moving cattle into their home pen establishes the caregiver as the provider of food and water. The bunk should be filled with grass hay and ration and the water tank filled with clean water before cattle arrival to encourage immediate nourishment and rehydration.

It is worthwhile to follow cattle into their home pen and move across the bottom third of the pen parallel to the bunk, allowing cattle to use their peripheral vision to view the

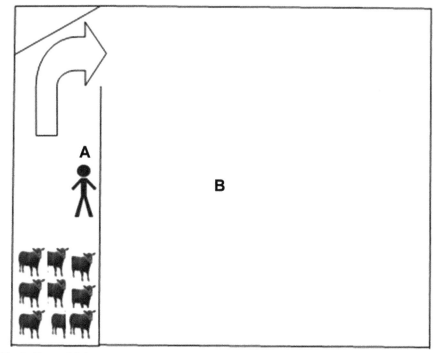

Fig. 2. To establish trust and provide guidance, the handler should be positioned at location A or B depending on the sensitivity of the cattle.

handler. Cattle ideally begin consuming food and water and may be left alone for the time being. In situations in which cattle do not go to or remain at the bunk, a caregiver who has followed the cattle into the pen is in the appropriate position to work with those animals. Cattle that lack trust in their handlers initially circle around handlers and avoid straight motion. The presence of the caregiver in the pen influences the herd to gather in a preferential corner. It is the handler's responsibility to use position, stimulus, and release to guide the herd to each corner of the pen. Moving cattle to each corner of the pen introduces them to the entirety of their new space; this is accomplished by working in a small square within the center of the pen. The handler should initially be orientated at a 45° angle to the corner where cattle are gathered (**Fig. 3**).

Cattle attention on the handler is necessary before motion within the group can be created. Uniform attention or alignment of the cattle is achieved by lateral movements of the handler parallel to the front of the group (**Fig. 4**). Once alignment is achieved, the group should be surveyed by the handler to identify the individual animals requesting guidance through their posture (**Fig. 5**). These animals are the front of the herd. The posture described is an animal standing broadside bending its neck to view the handler (**Fig. 6**).

Learning how to perpetuate straight motion is the key to guiding the front of the herd. Once the handler moves to a spot that allows the guidance-seeking animal to straighten its neck, the handler simply moves straight past the near-side eye. This handler movement encourages that animal to step forward. Once cattle motion is initiated, the handler should back up in a divergent line at a 45° angle with the motion of the cattle. This handler movement maintains motion by guiding the front animals and releasing pressure on the timid herd mates, allowing them to follow the leaders (**Fig. 7**).

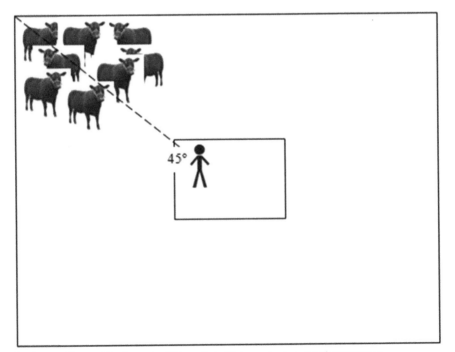

Fig. 3. Handler positioning at a 45° angle initiates voluntary herd movement.

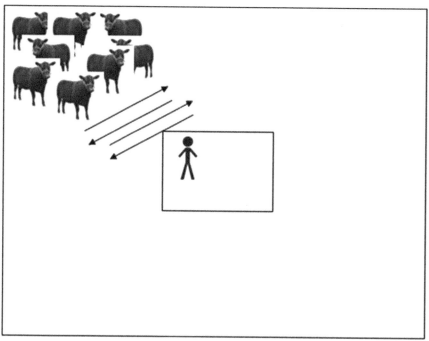

Fig. 4. The handler moves back and forth across the front of the herd at gentle angles to establish uniform alignment.

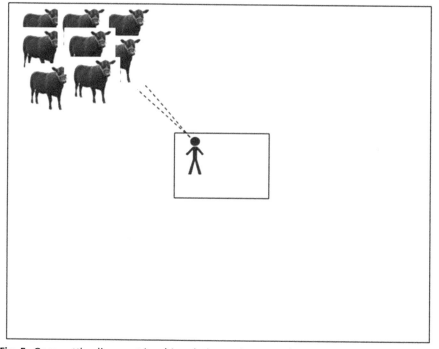

Fig. 5. Once cattle alignment is achieved, the cattle are ready to move as a unit.

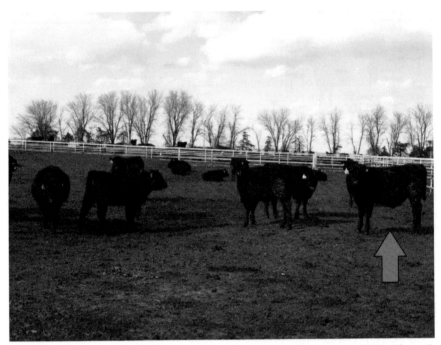

Fig. 6. The animal on the far right (*arrow*) is requesting guidance and visibility from the handler.

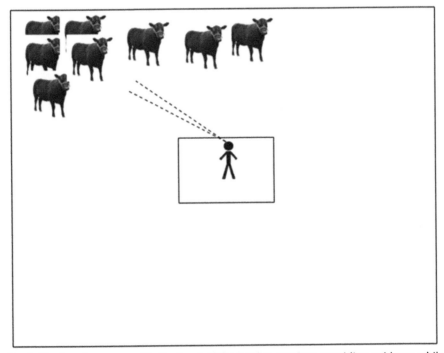

Fig. 7. The handler moves with the front of the herd to continue providing guidance while releasing pressure on timid animals at the back of the herd.

Once animals are willing to travel in a straight line from corner to corner around the pen, the handler can choose to leave the cattle at the bunk (**Fig. 8**). Pressure is applied in the back corner of the pen and released as the cattle arrive at the bunk area, encouraging bunk confidence.

A completely calm and confident herd does not develop with a single training session. Multiple sessions are needed over several days, and multiple training sessions within a single day are encouraged for new arrivals. Initially, training sessions should not be longer than 7 to 9 minutes because cattle become overwhelmed and the training becomes ineffective. Breaks lasting 30 minutes to several hours should be taken when cattle start to show fatigue. Indications that cattle are becoming tired are cattle lose focus on the handler, leaders are difficult to identify, and cattle stop motion more often. Training sessions should occur regularly for the first week after arrival. The sessions become longer than 7 to 9 minutes as cattle gain trust in the handler and decrease in length again when the group is consistently willing to work for the handler.

CONTINUED BENEFITS OF ACCLIMATION

Pen riders are responsible for continued acclimation throughout the feeding period. These are the individuals who interact with cattle on a daily basis. Being able to create orderly motion within a pen allows for systematic evaluation of every animal in the pen. When cattle trust their pen rider, sick animals reveal their true state of health and may walk by the pen rider for evaluation. Proper acclimation makes it easier and safer to pull an individual from a pen. Animals that trust their caregiver are more willing to leave the company of their herd mates.

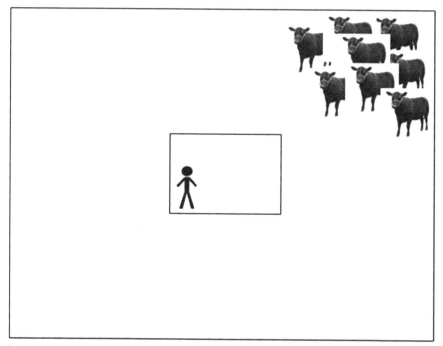

Fig. 8. The handler can either ask cattle to return to the corner they came from or preferably continue around the pen.

When cattle have been taught to work for their handlers, they are willing to pass by their handlers in an orderly fashion. This action allows cattle to be safely counted, sorted, or processed. As part of the acclimation process, cattle can be taught to move to and through the processing barn. Emptying the home pen and allowing cattle to move toward the processing barn without actually going to the barn teaches cattle that they can leave their home pen without having something done to them. This understanding makes cattle more willing to go to the processing barn at the time of processing. If time permits, cattle can be introduced to the processing facility by allowing them to move through the facility without being processed, which further encourages their cooperation at the time of processing.

Correctly emptying home pens reinforces acclimation training and prepares cattle for single file movement during processing, sorting, and loading. If possible, handlers should work in teams of 2 or 3 to empty a pen. As when emptying a holding pen, handlers should work from the side of the gate that allows cattle to maintain visualization of both the handler and their destination. When entering the pen to be emptied, handlers should remain calm and move through the herd asking the resting animals to stand up; this focuses the cattle's attention on the handlers. One handler should be positioned by the gate, whereas the other supports motion further back in the herd. The handler at the gate locates the leader of the group and then asks that animal to step forward by first moving to straighten the animal's head and then moving toward his ear, applying pressure at a 45° angle. The handler applies pressure to the other animals in a similar manner until orderly flow is established and then backs up and allows motion to continue. Any stray animals can be gathered after most of the pen has been emptied by asking them to follow the remainder of the herd.

Safety is the top priority each time caregivers interact with cattle. It is important for handlers not to position themselves without an escape route. A handler should never be inside a solid-walled tub with cattle or behind them in the snake (the single file alley to the chute). Caregivers should never be in a position to fail in terms of human and animal safety. In challenging environments, it is important for caregivers and pen riders to know their limitations and ask for assistance. Challenging environments can include pens with obstacles such as manure piles, hay bales, hills, or a large pen area where it is difficult for a single individual to maintain eye contact with cattle. Having multiple people allows eye contact to be maintained.

PROCESSING

Processing is the initial induction of new arrivals into the feedlot, typically scheduled 2 to 3 days after arrival. The goals of processing are to improve cattle health, increase performance, and continue training cattle. Activities involved in processing can include identification, parasite control, vaccination, hormone implantation, pregnancy management, and treatment if necessary. Veterinarians differ in their recommendations as to which actions are required for new arrivals. Gathering proper history on the cattle aids in making the best decisions for each group.

Cattle risk category has the largest impact on specific recommendations for a new group of cattle. In a survey of feedlot consultant veterinarians, cattle risk category was deemed the most critical factor in predicting cattle health.[18] Risk category is influenced by cattle origin, castration status and method, heifer pregnancy status, transit time, weaning status and method, vaccination history including dates and products, implant history, previous antibiotic usage, and any previous health problems. As such, great effort should be made by the feedlot manager to gather this information on new arrivals. A sample questionnaire form is shown in **Fig. 9**. Knowing the history of new arrivals allows producers to implement a targeted, cost-effective intervention strategy.

Cattle coming from a single source are at a decreased risk compared with those coming from multiple sources in which they are highly commingled. Single-source

Cattle Procurement History Form

Origin: Salebarn   Multiple Sources   Ranch   Single Source

Geographic Location:_____

Expected Transit Time:_____

Date Weaned and Method:

_____

Castration Status and Method:

_____

Heifers:

Pregnant   Guaranteed Open   Spayed   Unknown   Bull-Exposure

Dates of Bull-Exposure and Additional Comments:

_____

History of Implants: Yes   No

If Yes: Brand:_____   Date:_____

Vaccination History:

Respiratory Viruses: Yes   No

Date(s): _____   Product: _____

Pasturella Products: Yes   No

Date(s): _____   Product:_____

7-Way/Clostridial Products: Yes   No

Date(s): _____   Product:_____

Autogenous Vaccine: Yes   No

Date(s): _____   Organism:_____

Anthelminthic Usage: Yes   No

Date: _____   Product:_____

Antibiotic Usage: Yes   No

Date:_____   Product:_____

Health Comments:

Fig. 9. This document guides purchase interviews to gather cattle history.

cattle have established the social fabric of the herd and had uniform exposure to pathogens, whereas cattle from multiple sources do not have an established social hierarchy and can be introduced to new pathogens, increasing the risk of disease in the herd. In addition, purchase through a sale barn increases stress and places cattle in a higher risk category. A study performed in Australian feedlots tracked the mixing of individual animals before their induction into a feedlot. They found that mixing of cattle less than 12 days before entering a feedlot increased risk of BRD. However, mixing of cattle more than 27 days before entry to the feedlot was protective for BRD. Mixing 4 or more groups of cattle and moving through a sale yard within 12 days before arrival at the feedlot both increased BRD risk.[19]

Castration and pregnancy status affect how a group of animals is managed. Multiple studies have shown a decrease in ADG and an increase in morbidity when calves are castrated after arrival.[20] Thus, animals that require castration postarrival are placed in a higher risk category than steers. Post-arrival castration methods differ with weight class and facilities available. Similarly, pregnancy decreases ADG, as energy is diverted to pregnancy requirements instead of growth. Many feedlot managers choose to abort pregnant heifers, despite the associated costs. Knowing the castration and pregnancy status of arrivals allows proper processing plans to be implemented according to the appropriate risk category.

Another factor affecting risk category is transit time. Transit time, including marketing, can affect the health status of the animal as explained earlier relative to hydration, nutritional status, and cortisol levels. The Australian study tracking BRD risk factors found a greater risk for BRD in cattle that were transported more than 6 hours compared with those transported less than 6 hours.[19] The implications of changes in climate and geography from origin to destination varies with season. Cattle that experience a drastic climate change are at a greater risk for disease than those that remain in a similar climate. Research performed on cattle transport climates has shown that temperatures and microclimates within trailers can vary between $-42°C$ and $45°C$, which extends beyond the thermal neutral zone for cattle,[21–23] and this has been shown to negatively affect animal welfare.

Preconditioning has been promoted to reduce risk of BRD in cattle. Some preconditioning programs include only weaning, whereas others incorporate vaccination, dehorning, and castration. Regardless, multiple studies have shown preconditioning to reduce BRD morbidity in feedlots, with the greatest effect being attributable to weaning.[24] Weaning method should be considered when assigning risk category. Step and colleagues[25] evaluated the effect of weaning and immediate shipment compared with weaning, with or without vaccination, and remaining on the ranch for 45 days before shipment. Calves with unknown histories were purchased from market sources to serve as a control group. The study found that calves that remained on the ranch for 45 days postweaning had reduced morbidity compared with calves that were immediately shipped or calves purchased from a market source. A pilot study by Dewell and colleagues[26] provides preliminary evidence that acclimation and low-stress cattle handling may be associated with performance benefits when applied to abruptly weaned calves in a feedlot. Another study by Fell and colleagues[27] evaluated the effect of 3 methods of weaning (yard weaning, yard training, and paddock weaning) on the ADG of feedlot cattle. Yard weaning is a method of weaning in which cattle receive some handler interaction on a daily basis; this interaction is lacking in paddock weaning. Yard training involved teaching the animals to eat out of a bunk and drink from a trough. The investigators found yard-weaned and yard-trained cattle to have higher ADG than paddock-weaned cattle. In addition, they found the highest weight gains in calves that were yard weaned and vaccinated. It is evident from these studies that preconditioning has benefits in reducing BRD morbidity and reducing economic costs to producers. As such, animals that are preconditioned are at a lower risk than those that have not been preconditioned.

Age and vaccination status influence the presence of antibodies in cattle and are therefore important in assigning risk category. Scientific reasoning indicates that vaccinating before antigen exposure with adequate time for antibody development should provide greater protection than later vaccination. Cattle are at the greatest risk during the transition from passive immunity, when they rely on maternal antibodies, to active immunity, when they rely on their own antibody production. Thus, cattle arriving at the feedlot during this immune status transition are more susceptible to disease. A study by Lonergan[28] found that for each 45.4 kg decrease in arrival weight, mortality rates attributable to BRD increased 20% to 30%. A main factor contributing to failure in response to vaccination is an increased level of stress in animals on arrival at the feedlot. By vaccinating before arrival, stressors can be spaced out, increasing the likelihood of appropriate vaccine response.[24]

Although vaccination is common in the beef industry, evidence supporting the practice is limited. Taylor and colleagues[24] noted that, although research has shown antibodies to be protective against disease, other studies have found the antibodies produced in response to vaccine exposure are not always protective. Still, vaccination may help improve performance, and evidence-based medicine indicates vaccination of animals in commercial feedlots can reduce morbidity and mortality. The type of vaccine used affects the antibody response and duration of antibodies, with modified live vaccines having the greatest duration of antibody response.[29] A study by Step and colleagues[25] found an increase in the arrival weight of calves that were vaccinated at the time of weaning and remained on the ranch for 45 days before induction into the feedlot. Another study conducted on recently weaned beef calves in a Portuguese feedlot found 3% morbidity and 0% mortality in the group vaccinated at the feedlot with a multivalent BRD vaccine compared with 14% morbidity and 4% mortality in the unvaccinated group. The odds of getting BRD were 4.822 times greater in the unvaccinated group compared with the vaccinated group.[30] In a survey of 23 feedlot consultants, nearly all consultants recommended vaccination for infectious bovine rhinotracheitis (IBR) and bovine viral diarrhea virus (BVDV), and more than 50% recommended including vaccination for bovine respiratory syncytial virus (BRSV), parainfluenza 3 virus (PI3), and clostridial bacterin-toxoids.[18] Clostridial diseases cause sporadic death loss in feedlot environments. Without documentation of 2 prior doses of appropriate clostridial vaccine, feedlot managers should consider including a multivalent clostridial vaccine at processing.

Metaphylaxis is often executed at the time of processing. At present, 95% of feedlot consultants recommend metaphylaxis in high-risk cattle.[18] Metaphylaxis has been argued for because individual sick animals are difficult to identify, it is preventative as well as therapeutic for those already experiencing disease at the time of arrival, and it improves ADG while reducing BRD morbidity and mortality.[31] Those in opposition to metaphylaxis argue that acclimation can improve individual animal detection, and there is growing pressure from consumers for more judicious use of antibiotics. Ultimately, the decision to use metaphylaxis in a group of new arrivals needs to be based on cattle risk category, cost analysis of treatment, and a determination if metaphylactic treatment will improve cattle health and welfare.

Anthelminthics are commonly applied to all cattle at processing to aid in parasite control. It has been shown that strategic deworming can increase weight gain in animals both on pasture and after entry into the feedlot. Not only was ADG improved but feed efficiency was also improved for steers that had been dewormed compared with those not receiving fenbendazole.[32] In a survey of feedlot consultants, most preferred injectable parasiticides only.[18] Studies by Reinhardt and colleagues[33] showed that treatment with oral fenbendazole and ivermectin pour-on together was associated with reduced parasites and improved performance when compared with treatment with either a pour-on ivermectin or injectable dormectin alone. The management team must determine the best course of action for each arrival group.

Hormone implantation is a main component of processing new arrivals. Implants are intended to increase average rate of gain and feed conversion; they do so by increasing circulating levels of insulinlike growth factor-1 (IGF-1) and by stimulating cellular production of protein. IGF-1 stimulates production and differentiation of cells, whereas trenbolone acetate (an anabolic agent) stimulates protein production and decreases the catabolism of protein through reduction of ACTH levels.[34] The manager, nutritionist, and veterinarian should be involved in developing the implant program. The manager's goals for carcass quality and grade and prior implant usage are important considerations when choosing the most effective implant program for each group of cattle. The nutritionist's feeding program determines when hormone levels need to be adjusted for each phase of the feeding period. The veterinarian is often responsible for training the processing crew on proper placement of implants.[35] A team approach to developing the implant program is necessary to maximize efficacy and efficiency.

Processing speed depends on cattle temperament, crew experience, and the specific activities involved, but implanting is the most time-consuming step because of the importance of proper placement in avoiding adverse effects.[34] Processing crews that use acclimation and low-stress handling methods can process cattle at a rate of up to 8 head per minute. Processing is a team effort. It is just as important for the persons bringing cattle to a Bud Box or tub to practice low-stress handling as it is for those working at the chute. Handlers sending cattle to a tub or Bud Box must focus on timing and draft size. Cattle should never be placed in the tub or Bud Box when the snake is full of cattle. The draft size (the number of cattle brought to the tub) is determined by how many cattle immediately fit into the snake. The goal of the handler is to create a steady flow of cattle through the system while minimizing the time cattle spend in the system.

Bringing a draft to the Bud Box or tub is a simple process when working from the front of the group. The handler asks the first 1 or 2 animals to pass by and then walks with those animals to relieve pressure on the remainder of the cattle, allowing them to follow (**Figs. 10–12**, Video 4). Once the appropriate number of cattle have followed, the handler can simply move across the alley at an angle to cut-off the remainder of the group (**Fig. 13**). This change in handler position stops cattle motion behind the handler while encouraging the draft to continue moving forward. The same principles used when emptying a holding pen apply when emptying cattle from a Bud Box. Moving cattle through a tub requires cattle to have adequate space to turn and find the snake. Direction can be provided by applying pressure past the animal's eye (from head to tail) and by moving a hand or arm in a gentle swaying motion as if directing traffic toward the snake. Moving cattle through a snake requires the handler to work from the animal's head and move past their eye toward the tail. The animal moves away from this handler motion. Cattle attitude during processing can be measured by observing behaviors including vocalization, chute exit attitude, and speed of exit from the chute. This exit behavior is a function of facility design and handler expertise.

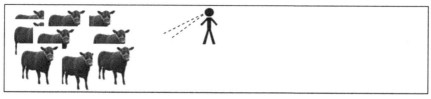

Fig. 10. The handler initiates cattle movement from the front of the group.

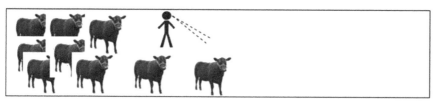

Fig. 11. The handler must ensure that the first 2 animals continue toward the Bud Box.

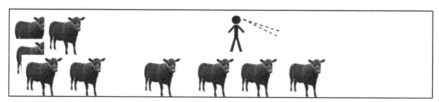

Fig. 12. Orderly motion in the front cattle draws additional cattle into the draft.

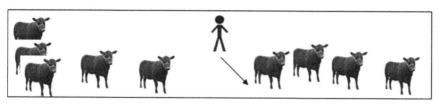

Fig. 13. Handler movement can stop flow of additional animals while maintaining their alignment for bringing the next draft.

SUMMARY

Acclimation procedures combined with proper processing of newly arrived cattle promote cattle well-being and performance from the day cattle arrive at the feedlot to the end of their feeding period. Spending time performing acclimation lessons with new arrivals reestablishes the social fabric of the herd; trains cattle to be confident; reduces stress; encourages rehydration, nourishment, and rest; and supports immune function. Furthermore, confident cattle are more likely to reveal their true state of health to those individuals who understand cattle communication, allowing for timely identification and treatment of disease and injury. Acclimation procedures also improve safety for both caregivers and cattle. A sound processing protocol and proper handling during processing can improve the effectiveness of products administered during initial processing, promoting health and well-being throughout the feeding period.

SUPPLEMENTARY DATA

Supplementary data related to this article can be found online at http://dx.doi.org/10.1016/j.cvfa.2015.06.002.

REFERENCES

1. Richeson JT, Pinedo PJ, Kegley EB, et al. Association of hematologic variables and castration status at the time of arrival at a research facility with the risk of bovine respiratory disease in beef calves. J Am Vet Med Assoc 2013;243(7): 1035–41.
2. Morgan SE. Water quality for cattle. Vet Clin North Am Food Anim Pract 2011; 27(2):285–95.
3. Brew MN, Carter J, Maddox MK. The impact of water quality on beef cattle health and performance. University of Florida: IFAS Extension; 2009. Publication #AN187. Available at: http://edis.ifas.ufl.edu/an187. Accessed April 19, 2015.
4. Faries FC Jr, Sweeten JM, Reagor JC. Water quality: its relationship to livestock. Texas A&M AgriLife Extension; 1998. Publication L-2374. Available at: https://repository.tamu.edu/bitstream/handle/1969.1/87665/pdf_370.pdf?sequence=1&isAllowed=y. Accessed April 19, 2015.
5. Brew MN, Myer RO, Hersom MJ, et al. Water intake and factors affecting water intake of growing beef cattle. Livest Sci 2011;140:297–300.
6. Preston RL. Receiving cattle nutrition. Vet Clin North Am Food Anim Pract 2007; 23:193–205.
7. Falkenberg SM, Carroll JA, Keisler DH, et al. Evaluation of the endocrine response of cattle during the relocation process. Livest Sci 2013;151:203–12.
8. Donovan DC, Hippen AR, Hurley DJ, et al. The role of acidogenic diets and ß-hydroxybutyate on lymphocyte proliferation and serum antibody response against bovine respiratory viruses in Holstein steers. J Anim Sci 2003;81:3088–94.
9. Calderon DF, Cook NB. The effect of lameness on the resting behavior and metabolic status of dairy cattle during the transition period in a freestall-housed dairy herd. J Dairy Sci 2011;94:2883–94.
10. Cooper MD, Arney DR, Phillips CJ. Two- or four-hour lying deprivation on the behavior of lactating dairy cows. J Dairy Sci 2007;90:1149–58.
11. Leonard FC, O'Connell JM, O'Farrell KJ. Effect of overcrowding on claw health in first-calved Friesian heifers. Br Vet J 1996;152(4):459–72.

12. Griffin D, Chengappa MM, Kuszak J, et al. Bacterial pathogens of the bovine respiratory disease complex. Vet Clin North Am Food Anim Pract 2010;26(2):381–94.
13. Frank GH. Bacteria as etiologic agents in bovine respiratory disease. In: Loan RW, editor. Bovine respiratory disease. College Station (TX): Texas A&M University Press; 1984. p. 347–62.
14. Srikumaran S, Kelling CL, Ambagala A. Immune evasion of pathogens of bovine respiratory disease complex. Anim Health Res Rev 2007;8(2):215–29.
15. Filion LG, Willson PJ, Bielefeldt-Ohmann H, et al. The possible role of stress in the induction of pneumonic pasteurellosis. Can J Comp Med 1984;48:268–74.
16. Buckham Sporer KR, Weber PS, Burton JL, et al. Transportation of young beef bulls alters circulating physiological parameters that may be effective biomarkers of stress. J Anim Sci 2008;86:1325–34.
17. Buckham Sporer KR, Burton JL, Earley B, et al. Transportation stress in young bulls alters expression of neutrophil genes important for the regulation of apoptosis, tissue remodeling, margination, and anti-bacterial function. Vet Immunol Immunopathol 2007;118:19–29.
18. Terrell SP, Thomson DU, Wileman BW, et al. A survey to describe current feeder cattle health and well-being program recommendations made by feedlot veterinary consultants in the United States and Canada. Bov Pract 2011;45(2):140–8.
19. Hay KE, Barnes TS, Morton JM, et al. Risk factors for bovine respiratory disease in Australian feedlot cattle: use of a causal diagram-informed approach to estimate effects of animal mixing and movements before feedlot entry. Prev Vet Med 2014;117:160–9.
20. Thomson DU, White BJ. Backgrounding beef cattle. Vet Clin North Am Food Anim Pract 2006;22:373–98.
21. Schwartzkopf-Genswein KS, Faucitano L, Dadgar S, et al. Road transport of cattle, swine and poultry in North America and its impact on animal welfare, carcass and meat quality: a review. Meat Sci 2012;92:227–43.
22. González LA, Schwartzkopf-Genswein KS, Bryan M, et al. Benchmarking study of industry practices during commercial long haul transport of cattle in Alberta, Canada. J Anim Sci 2012;90:3606–17.
23. Curtis SE. Assessing effective environmental temperature. In: Curtis SE, editor. Environmental management in animal agriculture. Ames (IA): Iowa State University Press; 1983. p. 71–7.
24. Taylor JD, Fulton RW, Lehenbauer TW, et al. The epidemiology of bovine respiratory disease: what is the evidence for preventive measures? Can Vet J 2010;51:1351–9.
25. Step DL, Krehbiel CR, DePra HA, et al. Effects of commingling beef calves from different sources and weaning protocols during a forty-two-day receiving period on performance and bovine respiratory disease. J Anim Sci 2008;86:3146–58.
26. Dewell GA, Dewell RD, Noffsinger T, et al. Impact of low stress cattle handling on calf health and performance. Proceedings of Academy of Veterinary Consultants Summer Meeting. Colorado Springs (CO), August 2–3, 2013.
27. Fell LR, Walker KH, Reddacliff LA, et al. Reducing feedlot costs by pre-boosting: A tool to improve the health and adaptability of feedlot cattle. Meat and Livestock Australia 2002. Available at: http://www.mla.com.au/Research-and-development/Search-RD-reports/RD-report-details/Productivity-On-Farm/Reducing-feedlot-costs-by-pre-boosting-A-tool-to-improve-the-health-and-adaptability-of-feedlot-cattle/1774. Accessed January 19, 2015.

28. Loneragan GH. Feedlot mortalities: Epidemiology, trends, classification. Proceedings of Academy of Veterinary Consultants Summer Meeting. Colorado Springs (CO), August 5–7, 2004.

29. Fulton RW, Confer AW, Burge LJ, et al. Antibody response by cattle after vaccination with commercial viral vaccines containing bovine herpesvirus-1, bovine viral diarrhea virus, parainfluenza-3 virus, and bovine respiratory syncytial virus immunogens and subsequent revaccination at day 140. Vaccine 1995;13(8):725–33.

30. Stilwell G, Matos M, Carolino N, et al. Effect of a quadrivalent vaccine against respiratory virus on the incidence of respiratory disease in weaned beef calves. Prev Vet Med 2008;85:151–7.

31. Nickell JS, White BJ. Metaphylactic antimicrobial therapy for bovine respiratory disease in stocker and feedlot cattle. Vet Clin North Am Food Anim Pract 2010;26:285–301.

32. Smith R, Rogers K, Huse S, et al. Pasture deworming and(or) subsequent feedlot deworming with fenbendazole (Safe-Guard®) I. Effects on grazing performance, feedlot performance, and carcass traits of yearling steers. Available at: http://www.safe-guardcattle.com/uploads/MOAT_OK1.pdf. Accessed February 26, 2015.

33. Reinhardt CD, Hutcheson JP, Nichols WT. A fenbendazole oral drench in addition to an ivermectin pour-on reduces parasite burden and improves feedlot and carcass performance of finishing heifers compared to endectocides alone. J Anim Sci 2006;84(8):2243–50.

34. FD Lehman, Rains JR. Implants: a valuable tool for the cattle feeding industry mechanism, strategy and technique. 1998. Available at: http://www.cabnr.unr.edu/resources/cattlemens/1998/01%20Raines.html. Accessed March 1, 2015.

35. Smith RA, Hollis LC. Interaction between consulting veterinarians and nutritionists in the feedlot. Vet Clin North Am Food Anim Pract 2007;23:171–5.

Use of Antimicrobial Metaphylaxis for the Control of Bovine Respiratory Disease in High-Risk Cattle

Samuel E. Ives, DVM, PhD*, John T. Richeson, PhD

KEYWORDS

- Bovine respiratory disease • Cattle • Control • Feedlot • Metaphylaxis • Stocker

KEY POINTS

- Despite decades of research, the prevalence and challenges associated with bovine respiratory disease (BRD) in stocker and feedlot operations remain.
- Preconditioned calves are better prepared to handle the transition from origin ranch to feedlot, yet there is incentive to purchase high-risk cattle at a reduced cost, which is influenced by the proven efficacy and availability of antimicrobial metaphylaxis.
- The poor sensitivity of current BRD field diagnostic methods, typical pathogenesis of BRD, and labor issues are additional reasons for use of metaphylaxis.
- Because of increased consumer concern surrounding antimicrobial use in food animals, practitioners should consider comprehensive and novel approaches to judiciously guide decisions on metaphylactic use of antimicrobials.

INTRODUCTION

It has been well documented that bovine respiratory disease (BRD) complex is the leading cause of morbidity and mortality in feedlot cattle.[1-3] Coupled with death loss, high treatment costs, decreased performance, and reduced carcass value, BRD leads to significant economic losses for cattle feeders.[4-7] The BRD syndrome is also one of the most extensively studied cattle diseases, with research beginning in the late 1800s and continuing today.[8] The US Library of Medicine Web site (PubMed) shows that from 1982 through April 29, 2009, there were 1952 publications on various aspects of bovine respiratory disease in that database.[9] Since 2009, there have been an additional 1070 publications related to BRD; however, the clinical impact of BRD continues to be a major concern.

The authors having nothing to disclose.
Department of Agricultural Sciences, College of Agriculture, Science and Engineering, West Texas A&M University, Box 60998, Canyon, TX 79016, USA
* Corresponding author.
E-mail address: sives@wtamu.edu

Over the years, multiple BRD symposiums have been held in an effort to bring together researchers, veterinarians, and industry members to review the latest in BRD research and to discuss future research needs. There are several common themes that have perpetuated throughout these symposiums and various other publications. From the published proceedings of the 1983 BRD symposium held in Amarillo, Texas, it was proposed that the true etiology of shipping fever (BRD) is the antiquated method that is used to market beef calves. Regarding the current beef marketing system, which has remained relatively unchanged for several decades, one could say that "we bring the cattle to the feed (ie, corn) rather than bringing the feed to the cattle." It has been estimated that the average number of middlemen between the rancher and the consumer is 15.[10] Similarly, it has also been suggested that 1 obstacle to the successful management of BRD in cattle populations is associated with the segmented infrastructure of the beef industry. Calves progress through the production phase, changing ownership at any and all points, which provides ample opportunity for pathogens associated with BRD to colonize the lower respiratory tract.[11] Calves entering the feedyard are often highly commingled from various sources, experiencing immunosuppression due to a multitude of stressors relative to the marketing process, and are susceptible to disease during the relocation process.

Although restructuring the beef production system would most likely reduce the incidence of BRD, this is not a realistic option for most producers, and overall beef production would likely decrease for alternative systems. The objective of this article is to serve as a practical guide for feedlot practitioners by addressing the importance of metaphylaxis and to address management considerations surrounding antimicrobial metaphylactic use.

THE IMPORTANCE OF ANTIMICROBIAL METAPHYLAXIS

Despite improved understanding of BRD and advancements in vaccine and antimicrobial technologies, the percentage of mortality associated with BRD has remained relatively unchanged.[12] Frequently advocated interventions in newly received feedlot cattle, such as vaccination against viruses or bacterial pathogens and nutritional manipulations, have been shown to have limited impact on the incidence of BRD.[8,13] However, the use of antimicrobial metaphylaxis upon feedlot arrival to cattle considered at high risk for development of clinical BRD signs has consistently been shown to reduce morbidity and mortality.[14–20] Metaphylaxis is defined as the treatment of an entire group or population of cattle with a US Food and Drug Administration (FDA)-approved antimicrobial with the intent of controlling the incidence of acute-onset disease in highly stressed, newly received calves.[21]

The etiology of BRD is multifactorial and often polymicrobial, with complex interactions among the host immune system, viral and bacterial pathogens, and the multiple phases of the beef production system resulting in environment, social and relocation challenges.[13,21,22] Accurate diagnosis is critical for effective treatment of disease; however, the nature of the BRD complex makes accurate case identification a challenging task for feedlot animal health technicians. Classical methods of diagnosis are based on visual observations of clinical signs including depression, anorexia, nasal and/or ocular discharge, lack of rumen fill, or respiratory signs such as coughing or labored breathing.[13,23,24] This method of diagnosis is subjective, and agreement between observers is often exceedingly divergent. Nevertheless, these clinical signs can be used to assign a semiobjective clinical illness score of 0 to 4 as defined by Perino and Apley (1998, **Table 1**).

Table 1		
Description of clinical illness scores		
Score	Description	Appearance
0	Normal	Normal
1	Slightly ill	Noticeable depression without apparent signs of weakness
2	Moderately ill	Marked depression with moderate signs of weakness without a significantly altered gait
3	Severely ill	Severe depression with signs of weakness such as significantly altered gait
4	Moribund	Moribund and unable to rise

Adapted from Perino LJ, Apley MD. Clinical trial design in feedlots. Vet Clin North Am Food Anim Pract 1998;14:356; with permission.

The final treatment decision often combines the clinical illness score with a determination of rectal temperature,[25] although temperature threshold values vary throughout the literature, ranging from at least 103°F[26] to at least 104.5°F.[27] These organized case definition methods are predominately used in research settings and are not as often utilized by feedlot personnel. In commercial feedlot production, decisions regarding prevention, control, and treatment regimens are outlined by the consulting veterinarian, and BRD treatment decisions are typically based on clinical observations, occasionally coupled with determination of rectal temperature.

Numerous studies have evaluated the effectiveness of clinical observations for the diagnosis of BRD based on pulmonary lesions evident at slaughter. Of 469 steers followed from birth to harvest, 35% received treatment for respiratory disease between birth and slaughter (29% percent exclusively during the feeding period), whereas 72% of the steers presented gross pulmonary lesions evident at slaughter. Furthermore, 68% of the steers with lesions evident were never treated for respiratory tract disease.[28] These results are similar to those of Tennant and colleagues[29] who found that of the 2336 head of cattle enrolled in the study, 83% possessed respiratory tract lesions and 59% possessed lung lesions and were never identified as ill or administered treatment. Thompson and others[30] also found that, of animals with lung lesions at slaughter, 69.5% had never been treated for BRD. Using a Bayesian analysis, it has been estimated that observations of clinical illness had a diagnostic sensitivity of 61.8% and specificity of 62.8%.[31] The results of these studies give a mere glimpse into the fallacies of the current state of BRD diagnosis. The limitations associated with BRD diagnosis largely contribute to the decision to use a metaphylactic antimicrobial strategy in place of subjectively identifying, pulling, and treating sick calves after arrival to a stocker or feedlot facility.

FACTORS THAT INFLUENCE THE DECISION TO USE METAPHYLAXIS

The innate and adaptive responses of a calf's immune system work together to prevent infection by decreasing adherence, migration, and proliferation of pathogens in the host, as well as mounting neutralizing humoral (antibody) responses against respiratory pathogens. The immune status and pathogen exposure of calves arriving to the feedlot varies greatly, and environmental factors and activities such as weaning, commingling, and transportation can negatively impact an animal's ability to fight infection.[32] Metaphylactic antimicrobial therapy is a tool that producers may use to improve animal health and performance in the absence of the ability to determine current disease status of an individual or a group of cattle.

Although determining the specific pathogen challenge present in newly arrived feedlot cattle is not practical, assessing the risk factors associated with the development of BRD may pose some value to managers and producers. Most commonly, metaphylactic treatment on arrival is used in situations in which the cattle are determined to be at high risk for BRD. Multiple studies have been conducted to evaluate the effects of predisposing factors that lead to the classification of cattle as high risk, yet there are few conclusive findings. The most widely accepted risk factor to calves is duration of shipping or transportation from the purchase origin to the feedlot destination.[33–35] Cattle are typically transported between 2 and 5 times throughout their lifetime, and the duration of transport may be associated with the degree of dehydration, physiologic stress, and environmental change. Other risk factors for the development of BRD include climatic variability or time of year that the cattle are received into the feedyard, the source and degree of commingling that has occurred prior to receiving, prior health/vaccination history, initial body weight, gender, disposition/temperament, and breed.[33,36] Generally, calves that are deemed as high risk are lightweight, recently weaned, highly commingled, or of auction market origin; additionally, they generally have experienced an extended transport time and have an unknown health/vaccination history. Furthermore, calves that are bulls at the time of arrival have a higher risk of BRD compared with steer cohorts.[37] This association is likely attributable to stress and trauma from the castration procedure itself, yet the castrate status upon arrival may also correlate with other preconditioning management procedures performed at the ranch of origin that are known to mitigate clinical BRD.[8]

Several biological methods have been studied and proposed to objectively predict BRD risk upon feedlot arrival and thus have potential to aid in the decision to use metaphylaxis for a particular individual or group of cattle. One such method is the use of hematological findings upon arrival,[37] and it was determined that cattle arriving with decreased eosinophil or increased red blood cell concentrations are at greater risk for subsequent development of clinical signs of BRD. Other studies have evaluated the ability of circulating concentrations of acute-phase proteins such as ceruloplasmin,[38] haptoglobin,[39] and serum amyloid-A[40] to predict or detect BRD with mixed results. Specifically, haptoglobin concentration has been reported to be useful for disease detection in 1 study,[41] but other studies[39,41] indicate that haptoglobin is limited in its use as a disease biomarker. Regardless of the efficacy of these proposed biological methods to better target BRD metaphylactic use or treatment, the procedure must be both cost-effective and timely for adoption to be considered in the commercial production setting.

PRICE DISCOVERY OF FEEDER CATTLE

Preconditioning programs have been used to improve health and value of calves around the time of weaning. Programs vary in intensity of protocol and range from solely a preweaning respiratory vaccination to a comprehensive protocol consisting of weaning, vaccinations, anthelmintic treatment, castration, dehorning, and feed bunk and water tank training for a minimum number of days prior to shipping. Ranch of origin vaccination protocols prepare calves immunologically before the pathogen challenges and stressors associated with shipping and commingling. Training reduces the stress of the move to a confinement feeding operation that often results in anorexia and dehydration for prolonged periods due to not understanding the new environment and associated social reorganization. Preconditioning studies have demonstrated the financial return to the cow–calf producer willing to invest the time and risk of the associated protocols.[42]

Comparatively, studies demonstrating returns for the cattle feeder purchasing preconditioned calves are rare. One study reported such returns from a commercial feedlot in Kansas.[43] Calves were procured from 2 auction barns in Kansas and Missouri with or without a history of preconditioning prior to sale and shipped to the feedlot. The calves with no preconditioning history had greater BRD morbidity, numerically greater mortality, reduced feeding performance, and increased days on feed. However, because the calves without a history of preconditioning were purchased for fewer dollars, they produced similar net return as those with a known preconditioning history. The authors believe that a thorough evaluation of cattle cost is necessary to define optimal return opportunities. Oftentimes, cattle considered at greater risk for BRD can be successfully managed with metaphylaxis upon arrival to greater net returns than preconditioned cattle because of lower purchase costs.

ANTIMICROBIALS APPROVED FOR METAPHYLACTIC USE

Currently, there are 8 injectable and 4 oral antimicrobials approved for metaphylactic use (**Table 2**) updated from an earlier publication.[11] It is not the intent of this article to review responses associated with each product but to add some general comments on the usage of feed, water, and injectable antimicrobials for controlling disease. Water medication use is limited in most feedlots due to the structure of the plumbing system that precludes treating individual pens of cattle. Large water tanks can be used, but the additional labor to assure continuous availability and proper dosing of drug administered via water limits use. Changes to the marketing of these products are currently under way by the FDA, and sponsors of the products and will be discussed.

Metaphylactic treatments administered through the feed are an option and offer the flexibility of timing of the dosing without the need for handling and restraint. Dosing of individual animals is affected by consumption of the medicated feed and can be troublesome, as animals experiencing BRD are often anorectic. Currently, 1 product (Pulmotil) is available only by veterinary feed directive (VFD) as a category 1 drug by the drug sponsor. The VFD stipulates a prescription by a licensed veterinarian of the product into a feed for a group of cattle after a veterinary-client-patient relationship has been established. As a category 1 drug, the medicated feed can only be manufactured by a feed mill that is licensed through the FDA from the type A article.[44] Once a VFD has been issued, the licensed feed mill may manufacture the product into a type B or C category product, and the herdsman may then offer it for treatment. The other oral products in **Table 2** are currently offered over-the-counter and do not require a VFD.

FDA Guidance 213[45] put into motion changes to all oral antimicrobial products administered through water or feed and currently available over the counter. The drug sponsors of each oral antimicrobial product have been asked to voluntarily remove any growth promotion claims and include VFD restrictions. It is understood that changes are under way to simplify the VFD and medicated feed manufacturing regulations, but they have not been published to date (May 2015). The once simple application of water and feed medications for metaphylactic treatment of BRD will be more onerous in the future, with the intention of regulators to improve stewardship of the available oral antimicrobials. Future use of oral medications in the feedlot is predicated on how user friendly the amended regulations appear.

MANAGEMENT BENEFITS OF METAPHYLAXIS

Since the last metaphylaxis update in 2011,[11] there have been several new additions to the injectable market for the control of BRD (see **Table 2**). Obviously, injectable products offer more accurate dosing of cattle compared with oral products, but

Table 2
Antimicrobials currently approved for the control of bovine respiratory disease

Trade Name	Drug Name	Label Indications (Related to BRD)	Route of Administration	Dosage
Advocin	Danofloxacin	For the control and treatment of BRD associated with M haemolytica and P multocida	Subcutaneous injection	2 mL/100 lb body weight
Aureo S 700	Chlortetracycline – sulfamethazine	As an aid in the maintenance of weight gains in the presence of respiratory disease such as shipping fever	Oral	350 mg/head/day
Aureomycin	Chlortetracycline	Control of bacterial pneumonia associated with shipping fever complex caused by Pasteurella subspecies susceptible to chlortetracycline	Oral	350 mg/hd/d
Baytril	Enrofloxacin	Treatment and control of respiratory disease in cattle at high risk of developing BRD associated with M haemolytica and P multocida, H somni, and M bovis	Subcutaneous injection	3.4–5.7 mL/100 lb body weight
Draxxin	Tulathromycin	Treatment and control of respiratory disease in cattle at high risk of developing BRD associated with M haemolytica and P multocida, H somni, and M bovis	Subcutaneous injection	1.1 mL/100 lb body weight
Excede	Ceftiofur	Treatment and control of BRD in cattle which are at high risk of developing BRD associated with M haemolytica and P multocida, and H somni	Subcutaneous injection at the base of the ear	1.5 mL/100 lb body weight
Micotil	Tilmicosin	Treatment of BRD associated with M haemolytica, P multocida and H somni; for the control of respiratory disease in cattle at high risk of developing BRD associated with M haemolytica	Subcutaneous injection	1.5–3 mL/100 lb body weight
Nuflor	Florfenicol	Treatment and control of respiratory disease in cattle at high risk of developing BRD associated with M haemolytica, P multocida, and H somni	Subcutaneous injection	6 mL/100 lb body weight
Pulmotil[a]	Tilmicosin	Control of BRD associated with M haemolytica, P multocida and H somni in groups of cattle, where active BRD has been diagnosed in at least 10% of the animals in the group	Oral	568–757 g/ton 100% dry matter
Terramycin	Oxytetracycline	Prevention and treatment of the early stages of shipping fever complex caused by P multocida susceptible to oxytetracycline	Oral	0.5–2 g/head/day
Zactran	Gamithromycin	Treatment of BRD associated with M haemolytica, P multocida, H somni and M bovis; control of BRD in cattle at high risk of developing BRD associated with M haemolytica and P multocida.	Subcutaneous injection	2 mL/110 lb body weight
Zuprevo	Tildipirosin	Treatment and control of respiratory disease in cattle at high risk of developing BRD associated with M haemolytica, P multocida, and H somni	Subcutaneous injection	1 mL/100 lb body weight

[a] Requires a VFD.

they have the disadvantage of an additional labor requirement and animal handling if used in an unanticipated BRD outbreak situation. Efficacy of antimicrobial products to control a severe BRD outbreak is not well documented, as this scenario is difficult to simulate in research.[46] Metaphylaxis is well accepted in lighter placements (<600 lb body weight) due to the lower cost of treatment per head and the perception that lighter cattle are at increased risk for BRD. Metaphylaxis in cattle over 600 pounds can be more intimidating because of the greater cost per head. Tennent and colleagues[29] reported that metaphylactic treatment on arrival in cattle averaging 715 pounds and considered at high risk of developing BRD significantly reduced morbidity, mortality, and increased carcass weights compared with those not treated upon arrival, leading to greater net returns. The authors of this article believe that a comprehensive analysis of disease risk, rather than initial body weight alone, should guide the decision to use metaphylaxis.

An opportunity overlooked at many cattle operations is the pharmacokinetic curve of the newer macrolide antimicrobials that offer several days of therapy above the minimum inhibitory concentration (MIC) for the BRD pathogens. This feature justifies the use of an extended postmetaphylactic interval (PMI), a concept where an efficacious drug is on board above the MIC of target bacterial pathogens in the lung, and the treated animals are not eligible for further antimicrobial treatment until the end of the interval. This concept has great application during the acclimation period of new arrivals to a stocker or feedlot operation. Instead of focusing resources on BRD detection during this critical arrival period, the focus can be on helping the cattle adapt to their new environment, feed, social structure, and daily activity with the cattle and feeding crews of the operation. Anecdotally, the authors have found that many animals that would otherwise be diagnosed and treated for BRD during the PMI period respond well staying with their pen mates and those, with severe clinical presentation can be moved to a less competitive environment with fewer animals and different feed. Most of these animals will return to their original pen without further antimicrobial treatment.

Another benefit of on-arrival metaphylaxis and the resulting PMI may be that it allows homeostatic conditions to return earlier in cattle, compared with pull and treat methods. Similar to BRD, stress-induced immune dysfunction in newly received cattle is highly complex, and extensive characterization of this phenomenon is outside the scope of this article. Nevertheless, increased cortisol synthesis in response to physical or psychological stressors can result in suppression of both innate and adaptive immune processes and therefore increase susceptibility to disease.[43] Disruption of the feedlot acclimation period via daily sorting, handling, and restraint of BRD diagnoses from a pen of newly received cattle is likely to prolong chronic stress conditions. Anecdotal observations suggest the feedlot acclimation period to be approximately 14 to 28 days, and this is substantiated in multiple cattle receiving studies that evaluated cortisol,[47,48] acute phase protein,[41] or hematological[47,49] concentrations periodically after arrival. Interestingly, the acclimation time course is similar to the recommended PMI for many of the long-acting macrolide antimicrobials available today. This may allow practitioners to rediscover and implement animal husbandry techniques during the PMI, rather than focusing on BRD diagnosis and treatment.

SUMMARY

Despite decades of research and increased availability of antimicrobials, the prevalence and challenges associated with BRD in stocker and feedlot operations remain. Preconditioned calves are better prepared to handle the transition from the origin ranch to the feedlot, yet there is incentive for buyers to purchase high-risk cattle at a reduced cost, and this is largely influenced by the proven efficacy and availability of antimicrobial metaphylaxis. The poor sensitivity of current BRD field diagnostic methods, typical pathogenesis of BRD, and labor issues are additional reasons for the use of metaphylaxis. Nevertheless, because of increased consumer concern surrounding antimicrobial use in food animals, practitioners should consider comprehensive and novel approaches to judiciously guide decisions on metaphylactic use of antimicrobials. These may include objective indices that consider multiple risk factor inputs and emerging research on biomarkers or other novel methods that may accurately assess the health risk of cattle.

ACKNOWLEDGMENT

The authors wish to thank Mrs Amanda Fuller for assistance in preparing this article.

REFERENCES

1. Woolums AR, Loneragan GH, Hawkins LL, et al. Baseline management practices and animal health data reported by US feedlots responding to a survey regarding acute interstitial pneumonia. Bov Pract 2005;39:116–24.
2. Edward AJ. Respiratory diseases of feedlot cattle in the central USA. Bov Pract 1996;30:5–7.
3. Smith RA. Impact of disease on feedlot performance: a review. J Anim Sci 1998; 76:272–4.
4. Griffin D. Economic impact associated with respiratory disease in beef cattle. Vet Clin North Am Food Anim Pract 1997;13:367–77.
5. Schneider MJ, Tait RG Jr, Busby WD, et al. An evaluation of bovine respiratory disease complex in feedlot cattle: impact on performance and carcass traits using treatment records and lung lesion scores. J Anim Sci 2009;87:1821–7.
6. Irsik M, Langemeire M, Schroeder T, et al. Estimating the effects of animal health on the performance of feedlot cattle. Bov Pract 2006;40:65–74.
7. Gardner BA, Dolezal HG, Bryant LK, et al. Health of finishing steers: effects on performance, carcass traits, and meat tenderness. J Anim Sci 1999;77:3168–75.
8. Taylor JD, Fulton RW, Lehenbauer TW, et al. The epidemiology of bovine respiratory disease: What is the evidence for preventative measures? Can Vet J 2010;51:1351–9.
9. Fulton RW. Bovine respiratory disease research (1983–2009). Anim Health Res Rev 2009;10:131–9.
10. Horton D. Management, marketing, and medicine. In: Loan R, editor. Bovine respiratory disease—a symposium. College Station (TX): Texas A&M University Press; 1984. p. 3–6.
11. Nickell JS, White BJ. Metaphylactic antimicrobial therapy for bovine respiratory disease in stocker and feedlot cattle. Vet Clin North Am Food Anim Pract 2010; 26:285–301.
12. Miles D. Overview of the North American beef cattle industry and the incidence of bovine respiratory disease (BRD). Anim Health Res Rev 2009;10:101–3.
13. Duff GC, Galyean ML. Board-invited review: recent advances in management of highly stressed, newly received feedlot cattle. J Anim Sci 2007;85:823–40.
14. Lofgreen GP. Mass medication in reducing shipping fever-bovine respiratory disease complex in highly stressed calves. J Anim Sci 1983;56:529–36.
15. Van Donkersgoed J. Meta-analysis of field trials of antimicrobial mass medication for prophylaxis of bovine respiratory disease in feedlot cattle. Can Vet J 1992;33: 785–95.

16. Frank GH, Briggs RE, Duff GC, et al. Effects of vaccination prior to transit and administration of florfenicol at time of arrival in a feedlot on the health of transported calves and detection of *Mannheimia haemolytica* in nasal secretions. Am J Vet Res 2002;63:251–6.
17. Guthrie CA, Rogers KC, Christmas RA, et al. Efficacy of metaphylactic tilmicosin for controlling bovine respiratory disease in high-risk northern feeder calves. Bov Pract 2004;38:46–53.
18. Cusack PMV. Effect of mass medication with antibiotics at feedlot entry on the health and growth rate of cattle destined for the Australian domestic market. Aust Vet J 2004;82:154–6.
19. Step DL, Engelken T, Romano C, et al. Evaluation of three antimicrobial regimens used as metaphylaxis in stocker calves at high risk of developing bovine respiratory disease. Vet Ther 2007;8:136–47.
20. Wellman NG, O'Connor AM. Meta-analysis of treatment of cattle with bovine respiratory disease with tulathromycin. J Vet Pharmacol Ther 2007;30:234–41.
21. Urban-Chmiel R, Grooms DL. Prevention and control of bovine respiratory disease. J Livestock Sci 2012;3:27–36.
22. Taylor JD, Fulton RW, Lehenbauer TW, et al. The epidemiology of bovine respiratory disease: What is the evidence for predisposing factors? Can Vet J 2010;51:1095–102.
23. Perino LJ, Apley MD. Clinical trial design in feedlots. Vet Clin North Am Food Anim Pract 1998;14:343–65.
24. Buhman MJ, Perino LJ, Galyean ML, et al. Association between changes in eating and drinking behaviors and respiratory tract disease in newly arrived calves at a feedlot. Am J Vet Res 2000;61:1163–8.
25. Thomson DU, White BJ. Backgrounding beef cattle. Vet Clin North Am Food Anim Pract 2006;22:373–98.
26. Fluharty FL, Loerch SC. Effects of dietary energy source and level on performance of newly arrived feedlot calves. J Anim Sci 1996;74:504–13.
27. Booker CW, Guichon PT, Jim GK, et al. Seroepidemiology of undifferentiated fever in feedlot calves in western Canada. Can Vet J 1999;40:40–8.
28. Wittum TE, Woolen NE, Perino LJ, et al. Relationships among treatment for respiratory tract disease, pulmonary lesions evident at slaughter and rate of weight gain in feedlot cattle. J Am Vet Med Assoc 1996;209:814–8.
29. Tennant TC, Ives SE, Harper LB, et al. Comparison of tulathromycin and tilmicosin on the prevalence and severity of bovine respiratory disease in feedlot cattle in association with feedlot performance, carcass characteristics, and economic factors. J Anim Sci 2014;92:5203–13.
30. Thompson PN, Stone A, Schultheiss WA. Use of treatment records and lung lesion scoring to estimate the effect of respiratory disease on growth during early and late finishing periods in South African feedlot cattle. J Anim Sci 2006;84:488–98.
31. White BJ, Renter DG. Bayesian estimation of the performance of clinical observations and harvest lung scores for diagnosing bovine respiratory disease in postweaned beef calves. J Vet Diagn Invest 2009;21:446–53.
32. Edwards TA. Control methods for bovine respiratory disease for feedlot cattle. Vet Clin North Am Food Anim Pract 2010;26:273–84.
33. Sanderson MW, Dargatz DA, Wagner BA. Risk factors for initial respiratory disease in United States' feedlots based on producer-collected daily morbidity counts. Can Vet J 2008;49:373–8.
34. Cernicchiaro N, White BJ, Renter DG, et al. Associations between the distance traveled from sale barns to commercial feedlots in the United States and overall

performance, risk of respiratory disease, and cumulative mortality in feeder cattle during 1997 to 2009. J Anim Sci 2012;90:1929–39.

35. Cole NA, Camp TH, Rowe LD, et al. Effect of transport on feeder calves. Am J Vet Res 1988;49:178–83.

36. Seeger JT, Grotelueschen DM, Stokka GL, et al. Comparison of feedlot health, nutritional performance, carcass characteristics and economic value of un-weaned beef calves with an unknown health history and weaned beef calves receiving various herd-of-origin health protocols. Bov Pract 2008;42:27–39.

37. Richeson JT, Pinedo PJ, Kegley EB, et al. Association of hematologic variables and castration status at the time of arrival at a research facility with the risk of bovine res-piratory disease in beef calves. J Am Vet Med Assoc 2013;243:1035–41.

38. Conner JG, Eckersall PD, Wiseman A, et al. Acute phase response in calves following infection with *Pasteurella haemolytica, Ostertagia ostertagi* and endo-toxin administration. Res Vet Sci 1989;47:203–7.

39. Burciaga-Robles LO, Holland BP, Step DL, et al. Evaluation of breath biomarkers and serum haptoglobin concentration for diagnosis of bovine respiratory disease in heifers newly arrived at a feedlot. Am J Vet Res 2009;70:1291–8.

40. Eckersall PD, Young FJ, McComb C, et al. Acute phase responses in serum and milk from dairy cows with clinical mastitis. Vet Rec 2001;148:35–41.

41. Richeson JT, Kegley EB, Powell JG, et al. Weaning management of newly received beef calves with or without continuous exposure to a persistently in-fected bovine viral diarrhea virus pen mate: Effects on rectal temperature and serum proinflammatory cytokine and haptoglobin concentrations. J Anim Sci 2012;91:1400–8.

42. Seeger JT, King ME, Grotelueschen DM, et al. Effect of management, marketing, and certified health programs on the sale price of beef calves sold through a livestock video auction service from 1995 through 2009. J Am Vet Med Assoc 2011;239:451–6.

43. Roth JA. Cortisol as a mediator of stress-associated immunosuppression in cattle . Animal Stress. New York: Springer; 1985. p. 225–43.

44. Animal Feed. Food and drug administration Web site. Available at: http://www.fda.gov/AnimalVeterinary/ResourcesforYou/ucm268129.htm#Veterinary_Feed_Directives. Accessed January 13, 2015.

45. Guidance for Industry #213. US Department of Health and Human Services, Food and Drug Administration, and Center for Veterinary Medicine. Available at: http://www.fda.gov/downloads/AnimalVeterinary/GuidanceComplianceEnforcement/GuidanceforIndustry/UCM299624.pdf. Accessed April 1, 2015.

46. Johnson JC, Bryson WL, Barringer S, et al. Evaluation of on-arrival versus promp-ted metaphylaxis regimens using ceftiofur crystalline free acid for feedlot heifers at risk of developing bovine respiratory disease. Vet Ther 2008;9:53–62.

47. Richeson JT, Kegley EB, Gadberry MS, et al. Effects of on-arrival versus delayed clostridial or modified live respiratory vaccinations on health, performance, bovine viral diarrhea virus type I titers, and stress and immune measures of newly received beef calves. J Anim Sci 2009;87:2409–18.

48. Gupta S, Early B, Ting STL, et al. Effect of repeated regrouping and relocation on the physiological, immunological, and hematological variables and performance of steers. J Anim Sci 2005;83:1948–58.

49. Richeson JT, Kegley EB, Powell JG, et al. Weaning management of newly received beef calves with or without continuous exposure to a persistently in-fected bovine viral diarrhea virus pen mate: Effects on health, performance, bovine viral diarrhea virus titers, and peripheral blood leukocytes. J Anim Sci 2012;90:1972–85.

A Systematic Review of Bovine Respiratory Disease Diagnosis Focused on Diagnostic Confirmation, Early Detection, and Prediction of Unfavorable Outcomes in Feedlot Cattle

CrossMark

Barbara Wolfger, DVM, PhD[a],*, Edouard Timsit, DVM, PhD[a],
Brad J. White, DVM, MS[b], Karin Orsel, DVM, MSc, PhD[a]

KEYWORDS

- Bovine respiratory disease • Feedlot • Detection • Health monitoring system
- Diagnostic test

KEY POINTS

- Serum haptoglobin concentrations are useful to confirm bovine respiratory disease (BRD) but several other parameters are not useful or need further research.
- Feed intake measurements, changes in cattle behavior, infrared thermography, and reticulorumen boluses have been successfully used for early disease detection.
- Prognostic methods using routinely collected treatment and cohort data at the time of treatment can be used to identify cattle at risk of unfavorable outcome.

INTRODUCTION

Despite substantial advances in antibiotics and vaccines against respiratory pathogens, bovine respiratory disease (BRD) remains the most common and economically important disease in the modern feedlot industry. Approximately 21% and 9% of cattle arriving with a bodyweight of less than 318 kg and at least 318 kg, respectively, are

The authors have nothing to disclose.
[a] Department of Production Animal Health, Faculty of Veterinary Medicine, University of Calgary, 3330 Hospital Drive Northwest, Calgary, Alberta T2N-4N1, Canada; [b] Department of Clinical Sciences, Kansas State University, Mosier Hall Q 211, 1800 Denison Avenue, Manhattan, KS 66506, USA
* Corresponding author.
E-mail address: bwolfger@ucalgary.ca

affected by BRD during the feeding phase.[1] The detrimental economic effects of BRD increase with disease severity and the number of treatments administered.[2–5]

Traditionally, feedlot personnel evaluate cattle health subjectively based on cattle behavior and appearance, which have limited sensitivity (62%) for detecting BRD.[6] One of the diagnostic challenges is the natural behavioral pattern cattle express in response to human presence, because as prey animals, cattle mask signs of weakness and disease.[7] Cattle with BRD are therefore often detected late in the disease process or not detected at all.[8] Nonetheless, early intervention is key to effective BRD treatment resulting in lower relapse rates and lower mortality.[9,10]

Furthermore, clinical signs expressed by sick animals are often not specific of BRD (ie, depression, loss of appetite, respiratory character change, and increased rectal temperature [DART]).[11] Consequently, a large proportion of treated cattle is not truly affected by BRD (specificity of clinical diagnosis = 63%).[6] An increase in specificity of BRD diagnosis would lead to more prudent use of antimicrobials and lower costs of BRD control in feedlots.[12]

Although widely used, treatment records using DART signs are poorly correlated with post-therapeutic prognosis.[13] Accurate prognosis of BRD at the time of treatment is crucial for effective management (drug selection, sorting). To improve accuracy of diagnosis, early detection, and prognosis of BRD, new methods and technologies have been developed recently . The objective of the current review is to provide a summary of BRD confirmatory diagnostic tests, early detection methods and modalities to estimate post-therapeutic prognosis or predict unfavorable or fatal outcomes by means of a rapid systematic review.[14]

METHODS
Definitions for the Search

The systematic review included confirmation, early disease detection, and modalities to estimate post-therapeutic prognosis or predict unfavorable or fatal outcomes of BRD. Definitions for outcomes included in the review are as follows:

1. The case definition of BRD in the included manuscripts has to be based on a minimum of clinical signs of respiratory disease and elevated rectal temperature (threshold varied among studies, but $\geq 39.5°C$).
2. Confirmatory tests are laboratory and other tests used to increase specificity of BRD case definition.
3. Early disease detection methods are those used to detect sick cattle before obvious visual signs of BRD appear.
4. Prognostic methods at the time of initial treatment identify cattle at risk for multiple treatments or unfavorable outcome.

Criteria for Considering Studies

The review question was defined based on key concepts in terms of population (P), intervention (I), comparator (C), outcome (O) and study design (S), as described in the PRISMA statement.[15] The population of interest for this review was newly arrived feedlot calves. Studies were considered if they included beef breeds at the age of weaning (6–9 mo) up to yearlings (11–12 mo).[16] The purpose of the article was not to look for interventions or risk factors, but rather methods and technologies to detect and diagnose BRD and provide a post-therapeutic prognostic outcome. The comparator was the current industry standard. Studies were included if they used visual detection methods and at least hyperthermia ($\geq 39.5°C$). Outcomes of interest were confirmatory, early detection, or prognostic means to evaluate the efficacy of the method or technology. All study designs were considered for this review.

Search Strategy

Owing to the scope of the study (rapid systematic review), only studies in English published in international peer-reviewed journals were considered. Studies of all available years were identified by electronic searches in the Commonwealth Agricultural Bureau (CAB) Abstracts and PubMed. The search strategy included the population, method, comparator and outcome (**Box 1**). A search combining individual terms with "AND" was used to identify relevant articles. Searches were performed in December 2014 and January 2015, with the last update on February 17, 2015.

Selection of Studies

One reviewer (B.W.) assessed titles and abstracts for eligibility. If the article seemed to be relevant, the same reviewer evaluated the full text of the manuscript for inclusion. Relevant studies described confirmation, early detection, and modalities to estimate post-therapeutic prognosis or predict unfavorable or fatal outcomes in naturally occurring or experimentally induced BRD. Only original studies were included. The data extraction process was performed by one individual (B.W.) and verified by a second reviewer (K.O.). With the large variability of methods, study designs and reported outcomes, we decided to report outcomes as a descriptive review.

RESULTS AND DISCUSSION

The literature search including evaluation of titles and abstracts identified 71 studies for full-text screening. After complete review of the manuscript, 42 were excluded for the following reasons: 2 described technique development; 23 presented an outcome that was not diagnostic confirmation, early detection related, or prognosis; 11 reported detection methods for single pathogens outside the context of BRD; 2 were review papers; 2 had no full-text available; and 2 described only chronic pneumonia. Twenty-nine remaining articles were used for analysis (**Fig. 1**), including 3 retrospective data analyses,[17–19] 7 case controls,[20–26] 1 cohort study,[27] 12 longitudinal studies,[8,28–38] 5 infection trials,[39–43] and 1 combined longitudinal and infection trial.[44]

Box 1
Search terms to extract manuscripts of interest. Rows were combined with AND

Feedlot*OR concentrated animal feeding operation OR CAFO* OR feeding unit OR finishing unit OR feed yard OR feedyard

Cattle OR calves OR bovine

Respirator* OR BRD* OR bovine respiratory disease OR shipping fever OR bronchopneumonia OR undifferentiated fever

Detect* OR diagnos* OR radio-frequency identification system OR RFID OR thermography OR reticulo-rumen temperature OR ruminal OR infection marker OR acute phase protein OR temperature OR accelerometer OR screen* OR eating behavior OR behavior OR behavior OR eating behavior OR feeding behavior

*Wildcard operator (enables retrieval of records with any character after the asterisks).

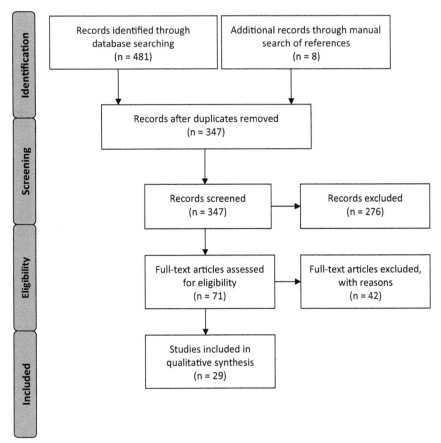

PRISMA 2009 Flow Diagram

Fig. 1. Stepwise exclusion of literature evaluated for inclusion in the rapid systematic review. (*From* Moher D, Liberati A, Tetzlaff J, et al. Preferred reporting items for systematic reviews and meta-analyses: the PRISMA Statement. Open Med 2009;3:e125.)

Part 1: Confirmatory Diagnostics

Confirmatory BRD diagnostics are tests that could be used to augment the visual observation, and typically would improve the specificity of diagnosis through the interpretation in series on only identified cases. The objective of this section was to review the available literature related to confirmatory diagnostic tests; therefore, many comparisons of test accuracy are made relative to visually identified cases. Caution should be taken when evaluating sensitivity and specificity of confirmatory tests because many were evaluated in comparison with only cases identified by visual observation and not the general population.

White blood cell count

White blood cell (WBC) count, specifically neutrophilia, left shift, neutropenia, lymphopenia, or increased neutrophil/lymphocyte ratio, has been used for decades to confirm mild to severe inflammation in cattle.[45] Based on an infection trial, exposure to persistently infected steers with bovine viral diarrhea virus resulted in significantly less WBC and neutrophils, whereas inoculation with *Mannheimia haemolytica* resulted in greater

WBC and neutrophils.[39] Lymphocyte count decreased with exposure to persistently infected animals and *M haemolytica*.[39] In another infection trial,[42] WBC and segmented neutrophils increased on day 1 after infection with *M haemolytica*, but decreased to baseline thereafter.

Neutrophil/lymphocyte ratio and WBC were compared with a clinical illness score and rectal temperature in naturally occurring BRD outbreaks.[33,34] In these studies, sensitivity and specificity for WBC ranged between 25% and 78% and between 80% and 94%, respectively. In a longitudinal study,[29] 52% of naturally occurring BRD had WBC and neutrophil counts greater than the laboratory provided reference range, and 20% had lymphocyte counts above or below the reference range. Given the wide range and often low accuracy compared with clinical signs, WBC, neutrophils, lymphocytes, and their respective ratios are of limited value to confirm BRD in feedlot cattle.

Acute phase proteins

Positive acute phase proteins (ie, haptoglobin [HAP], serum amyloid A, fibrinogen, apolipoprotein AI, and lipopolysaccharide binding protein [LBP]) are expected to increase in cattle with inflammation and tissue damage, whereas negative acute phase proteins (ie, transferrin) should decrease.[45] Changes in acute phase proteins have been associated with BRD in infection trials,[40,43] and naturally occurring BRD[24,29] (**Table 1**). On days 0.5, 1, 2, 3, and 7 after *M haemolytica* infection, HAP was increased in infected versus control cattle with no difference reported on day 9 after infection.[43] In an infection trial using bovine herpes virus 1 and *M haemolytica*, HAP and apolipoprotein AI were significantly increased by day 4 after viral exposure and before *M haemolytica* infection.[40]

Comparable results were reported in naturally occurring BRD outbreaks.[24,29] In a receiver-operator characteristics analysis comparing clinical illness to acute phase protein levels, both serum HAP (cutoff $\geq$0.81 mg/mL) and LBP ($\geq$0.33 µg/mL) levels were 93% sensitive. Specificity was 86% for HAP and 93% for LBP. In contrast, transferrin was not significantly lower in BRD cases compared with time-matched controls.[24] Furthermore, 94% of clinically sick cattle had HAP levels above the laboratory internal cutoff of 0.15 mg/mL and 76% had serum amyloid A levels above the cutoff (80.31 µg/mL).[29] It is noteworthy that cutoffs for HAP differ significantly between studies, which can be explained by the kits used (ie, Bovine Haptoglobin ELISA kit [Immunology Consultants Laboratories, Portland, OR[24]] vs Bovine HAP ELISA kit [Tridelta Development Ltd, Maynooth, Ireland[29]]). Given the results, HAP and potentially LBP can be used for laboratory confirmation of BRD, whereas limited evidence regarding other acute phase proteins currently hampers conclusions.

Detection of bovine respiratory disease pathogens

Establishing the presence of causative pathogens of BRD might aid in confirming BRD status, choice of treatment, and prophylactic methods such as targeted vaccination strategies. However, differentiation of BRD-affected cattle based on visual signs and hyperthermia ($\geq$40°C) from controls based on the respiratory flora is difficult.[26] *Pasteurella multocida* was isolated more frequently in cases than controls in nasal swabs (69% of cases and 46% of controls) and bronchoalveolar lavage (BAL; 68% of cases and 43% of controls), and *M haemolytica* was isolated more frequently in nasal swabs of controls (15% of cases and 32% of controls; no difference between cases and controls for BAL).[26] However, frequency of isolation of all other tested bacteria (*Mycoplasma bovis*, *Mycoplasma bovirhinitis*, and *Histophilus somni*) from the upper and lower respiratory tract was similar in cases versus controls.[26] Conversely,

Table 1
Acute phase protein changes during bovine respiratory disease (BRD) compared with controls (C) if not specified differently

Reference	Study Design	n	BRD	C	Outcome
Aich et al,[40] 2009	Infection trial (BHV-1 + M haemolytica)	20	6	14	HAP - ↑ day 4[a] (P<.05)
		—	—	—	Apolipoprotein AI - ↑ day 4[a] (P<.05)
Berry et al,[36] 2004	Longitudinal	245	64	45	HAP – treatment > recovery (P<.05)
Burciaga-Robles et al,[32] 2009	Longitudinal	337	222	42	HAP highest at initial treatment (P = .01)
Idoate et al,[24] 2015	Prospective case control	77	14	14	HAP treatment (cutoff: 0.81 mg/mL)
		—	—	—	Sensitivity = 92.9%
		—	—	—	Specificity = 85.7%
		—	—	—	LBP treatment (cutoff 0.33 µg/mL)
		—	—	—	Sensitivity = 92.9%
		—	—	—	Specificity = 92.9%
		—	—	—	Transferrin – ns
Purdy et al,[27] 2000	Cohort	101	73	28	HAP: diagnosis 2.36× >recovery
		—	—	—	Fibrinogen - ns
Theurer et al,[43] 2013	Infection trial (M haemolytica)	—	—	—	HAP - ↑ day 0.5–day 3[a] and day 7[a]
		—	—	—	HAP–matrix metalloproteinase-9 ↑ day 2-day 3[a]
Burciaga-Robles et al,[39] 2010	Infection trial (BVDV pi + M haemolytica)	24	18	6	HAP - ↑ 18–96 h[b]
Wolfger et al,[29] 2015	Longitudinal	213	66	48	Cases: 94% HAP pos.
		—	—	—	Cases: 75.4% SAA pos.

Abbreviations: BHV, bovine herpesvirus; BVDV, bovine viral diarrhea virus; HAP, haptoglobin; LBP, lipopolysaccharide binding protein; ns, not significant.
[a] Day relative to bacterial infection.
[b] Hour relative to bacterial infection.

a more recent study provided evidence for more frequent detection of *M haemolytica* in nasal swabs of cases (45%) compared with controls (28%), whereas *P multocida* was associated negatively with BRD (P<.02).[37] Therefore, clear differentiation between cases and controls on the basis of respiratory flora seems difficult.

Stress-related hormones
Cytokines stimulate the hypothalamic–pituitary–adrenal axis and increase peripheral glucocorticoid concentrations.[46] Substance P regulates nociceptive neurons and can be involved in pain, stress, and anxiety.[47] Blood cortisol concentrations have been measured in cattle to diagnose BRD.[33,34,43] Infected heifers had significantly higher serum concentrations of both cortisol and substance P immediately after *M haemolytica* infection (0.5–1 days after infection), but were not significantly different from control heifers on days 2 through 7, whereas substance P was lower on day 7 compared with uninfected control heifers.[43] In a natural BRD infection, serum cortisol concentration (>105.9 µmol/L) at the time of BRD diagnosis had a diagnostic sensitivity of 100%, but a specificity of only 53.8% compared with a disease definition including clinical illness score, WBC, neutrophil/lymphocyte ratio, and rectal temperature.[33] Salivary cortisol had a sensitivity of 70% and specificity of 52.9% in an earlier study conducted by the same research group.[34]

Elevated concentrations of cortisol are not specific to infection or inflammation and are elevated in common stress situations, which explains the low specificity of cortisol to diagnose BRD.[48] More evidence is needed to assess the diagnostic value of substance P in cattle with BRD.

Direct measurement of pulmonary changes

In addition to analyses of blood and clinical samples (nasal swabs and BAL), other analytical methods examining pulmonary changes have been proposed for BRD detection, but all seem to be of limited value.[23,25,32] Percutaneous lung biopsy was deemed easy to perform, but histopathologic changes were only observed in 17.9% of all successfully extracted lung samples collected from BRD cases.[23] Samples obtained by BAL detected inflammatory changes in the lower respiratory tract of both BRD cases and controls, with 35% of cases having normal differential cell counts.[25] Breath analysis of exhaled (e) CO, CO_2, and N_2O, and their respective ratios revealed that $eN_2O:eCO_2$ and $eCO:eCO2$ increased with number of treatments.[32] However, breath analysis in cattle remains experimental and further evaluation seems to be necessary before it can be recommended for confirmation of BRD.

Thoracic ultrasonography has been explored recently for BRD confirmation.[21,22] Ultrasonography identified lung lesions in 29% of BRD cases, 10% of arrival fever cases, and 16% of controls.[22] In contrast, a similar study evaluating 29 BRD cases and 15 controls reported significantly more sites with consolidation, pleural irregularities, maximal depth of consolidation, maximal area of consolidation, total consolidated area, and affected sites in BRD cases than controls ($P<.001$).[21] Based on contrasting results and limited sample sizes, we inferred that more studies are needed to evaluate the value of ultrasonography to confirm BRD. Current evidence is not conclusive to support the use of percutaneous lung biopsy, BAL, breath analysis, and ultrasonography to confirm BRD status in feedlot cattle.

Part 2: Early Disease Detection

Automated recording systems monitor cattle continuously without human presence. Therefore, this approach may increase the probability of identifying subtle changes of early or mild stages of disease that could be masked by cattle or not detectable by visual appraisal.[7]

Automated behavior monitoring

Evidence for differences in behavior between sick and healthy cattle Sick animals commonly decrease feeding and increase time of rest as a means to coordinate energy expenditure.[49] Output from location monitoring (Ubisense Series 7000 Compact Tag; Ubisense, Denver, CO) and accelerometers (GP1 SENSR; Reference LLC, Elkader, IA) provided evidence for differences in behavior between M haemolytica–infected heifers with mild symptoms of BRD and control heifers (**Fig. 2**).[43] However, there was no treatment effect on pedometer output (NL-800; New-Lifestyles Inc, Lees Summit, MO).[43] In another M haemolytica infection study using accelerometers, there were lower step counts ($P<.05$) and decreased standing time after inoculation compared with before infection.[42]

More evidence for the association among cattle behavior and disease status was provided in natural BRD outbreaks where individual feeding behavior (Growsafe, Airdrie, AB, Canada) was monitored. Sowell and colleagues[31] and Buhman and colleagues[30] reported shorter daily time at the feedbunk and less frequent visits 1 to 4 days on feed and 11 to 27 days on feed, respectively, for cattle with BRD compared with those that were visually healthy.

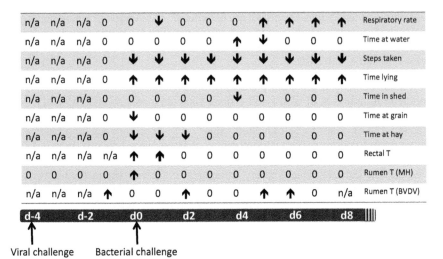

n/a	n/a	n/a	0	0	↓	0	0	0	↑	↑	↑	↑	Respiratory rate
n/a	n/a	n/a	0	0	0	0	0	↑	↓	0	0	0	Time at water
n/a	n/a	n/a	0	↓	↓	↓	↓	↓	↓	↓	↓	↓	Steps taken
n/a	n/a	n/a	0	↑	↑	↑	↑	↑	↑	↑	↑	↑	Time lying
n/a	n/a	n/a	0	0	0	0	0	↓	0	0	0	0	Time in shed
n/a	n/a	n/a	0	↓	0	0	0	0	0	0	0	0	Time at grain
n/a	n/a	n/a	0	↓	↓	↓	0	0	0	0	0	0	Time at hay
n/a	n/a	n/a	n/a	↑	↑	0	0	0	0	0	0	0	Rectal T
0	0	0	0	↑	0	0	0	0	0	0	0	0	Rumen T (MH)
n/a	n/a	n/a	↑	0	0	↑	0	0	↑	↑	0	n/a	Rumen T (BVDV)
d-4		**d-2**		**d0**		**d2**		**d4**		**d6**		**d8**	

↑ Viral challenge   ↑ Bacterial challenge

Fig. 2. Clinical and behavioral signs change after viral and bacterial infection. (*Data from* Refs.[40–43])

Application for early bovine respiratory disease detection Knowledge regarding different feeding patterns in healthy and sick cattle was used to identify BRD-affected cattle earlier than visual appraisal (**Fig. 3**). Using a cumulative sum chart of automatically collected feeding time, 85% and 96% of cattle with visual BRD signs were predicted on average 4.5 days before visual detection.[20] Further development

Sensitivity	61	78	82	77	81	81	80	Feed intake[29]
Specificity	84	79	78	77	77	77	79	
Sensitivity	69	59	77	71	81	77	75	Feeding time[29]
Specificity	83	80	79	78	78	76	79	
Sensitivity	n/a	54	54	54	n/a	n/a	n/a	IRT absolute[34]
Specificity		68	68	68				
Sensitivity	n/a	69	69	69	n/a	n/a	n/a	IRT ratio[34]
Specificity		77	77	77				
Sensitivity	n/a	81	81	81	n/a	n/a	n/a	Salivary cortisol[34]
Specificity		53	53	53				
Sensitivity	n/a	62	62	62	n/a	n/a	n/a	White blood cell count[34]
Specificity		77	77	77				
Sensitivity	n/a	46	46	46	n/a	n/a	n/a	Neutro/Lympho ratio[34]
Specificity		68	68	68				
	d-6		**d-4**		**d-2**		**d0**	

↑ Visual signs

Fig. 3. Sensitivity and specificity (%) of laboratory, clinical and behavioral parameters before visual detection (d_0). Infrared thermography (IRT) measured as absolute (orbital maximum value) and ratio (individual mean IRT maximum/mean infrared maximum of contemporary group); neutrophil–lymphocyte ratio (neutrophil/lymphocyte [neutro/lympho] ratio) measured as absolute neutrophil count/absolute lymphocyte count. n/a, not measured.

of the same technology measured intake during bunk visits. In a predictive algorithm, mean intake per meal, daily frequency of meals, and interval between meals identified BRD affected cattle up to 7 days before visual identification.[29] Furthermore, 60% to 81% of BRD cases were classified as sick, whereas 77% to 85% of visually healthy cattle were classified correctly between 1 and 7 days before visual identification.[29] Therefore, feeding behavior can be used to identify cattle before visual detection. Although promising in induced challenge trials, further studies are necessary to evaluate sensitivities and specificities of location monitoring systems, accelerometers, and pedometers for the use of early BRD detection in naturally occurring BRD.

Automated temperature measurements

Evidence for differences in temperature between sick and healthy cattle Based on expected changes in body temperature, several automated temperature measure devices have been applied for BRD detection: reticuloruminal boluses,[8,28] infrared thermography (IRT) measuring nasal passage and nasal planum surface[43] or radiated orbital temperature,[33,34] and temperature-sensing eartags measuring tympanic temperature.[44] Two *M haemolytica* infection trials reported altered body and surface temperatures after infection.[41,43] Average daily ruminal temperature (SmartStock LLC, Pawnee, OK) was only elevated on the day of *M haemolytica* challenge.[41] However, in a group of cattle housed with bovine viral diarrhea virus–persistently infected steers, hourly ruminal temperature was intermittently increased before and after *M haemolytica* infection (see **Fig. 2**).[41]

Nasal planum surface temperature measured by IRT (ThermaCAM S65, FLIR Systems, Wilsonville, OR) was higher in *M haemolytica* infected heifers at 8 and 48 hours after infection, and nasal passage temperature (Biothermal RFID Chip, Destron Technologies, Round Rock, TX) was lower between 14 and 18 hours after infection.[43] In naturally occurring BRD, maximum orbital temperature measured with IRT (FLIR Comp, Boston, MA), had a positive predictive value of 86% and a negative predictive value of 100% on the day of visual BRD identification.[33] In an earlier study, the same research team reported 87% positive predictive value and 67% negative predictive value on the day of visual BRD detection.[34]

The percentage of BRD-affected calves exceeding 39.8°C tympanic temperature (Fever Tags, Amarillo, TX) varied between 15% and 85% in a study that used several groups of newly arrived feedlot cattle.[44] Therefore, changes in body temperature associated with BRD can be measured reliably with IRT and reticulorumen boluses, whereas technology measuring tympanic temperature might need further development.

Application in early bovine respiratory disease detection Hyperthermia is one of the first signs of BRD, based on infection trials (see **Fig. 2**).[41,43] From 4 to 6 days before visual detection of naturally occurring BRD, maximum orbital temperature was 54% sensitive and 68% specific (see **Fig. 3**).[34] The ratio between individual mean temperature and the group orbital temperature increased sensitivity to 69% and specificity to 77%.[34] In another trial,[28] 73% of steers with reticulorumen hyperthermia lasting longer than 6 hours (Thermobolus, Medria SAS, Chateaugiron, France) in a naturally occurring BRD outbreak were subsequently confirmed as BRD cases (based on rectal temperature of ≥39.7°C and abnormal pulmonary sounds). The study additionally provided evidence that first clinical signs detectable by visual appraisal appear between 12 and 136 hours after hyperthermia.[28] Therefore, hyperthermia may provide first evidence of BRD in feedlot cattle, but further clinical evaluation of suspect animals is necessary to confirm BRD; because changes in body temperature are not only caused by BRD.

Part 3: Prognostic Tests

Chute-side tests at the time of treatment could help identify cattle at higher risk for unfavorable BRD outcome (ie, multiple treatments or death) and enable feedlot managers to manage those cattle more effectively. A better understanding of the expected prognosis at the time of therapy could influence treatment and subsequent management decisions.

Biomarkers and pathogen detection

Proteomic, metabolite, and serum elemental profiles (ie, minerals, trace elements) can be used to predict mortality. Elemental profiles (ie, Li, B, Mg, P, Ca, Ti, Cr, Fe, Cu, Zn, Se, Sr, Mo, Cd, and Ba), lower lactate concentrations and higher cortisol concentrations predicted mortality before viral infection.[40] In contrast, higher glucose concentrations 4 days after viral infection were associated with survival ($P<.05$).[40]

Although lactate concentrations could not predict fatal disease outcome at the time of BRD diagnosis in naturally occurring BRD, a 1-log increase in follow-up lactate concentrations (3, 6, 9, and 15 days after first treatment) increased the hazard of dying before the next observation by a factor of 36.5 (95% CI, 3.5–381.6).[35] Further studies are needed to assess the true prognostic nature of lactate. One study using pathogen detection showed that calves with a positive culture for M bovis on nasal swab at initial BRD treatment were more likely to die (odds ratio [OR], 3.0) or require a second (OR, 3.3) or third (OR, 3.2) treatment.[38] Detection of specific pathogens could be useful to predict unfavorable BRD outcomes, but more research is required to evaluate the influence of specific pathogens on case outcomes.

Direct indicators for lung lesions

Several methods have been used recently to identify lung lesions directly in BRD cases at the time of first identification. The methods described herein were described only in single published papers; therefore, no consensus of the potential impact can be evaluated from currently published literature.

A stethoscope that automatically assigns respiratory scores from 1 to 5 at first BRD identification (Whisper Veterinary Stethoscope, Plymouth, MN) predicted survival of BRD cases moderately (AUC = 0.64).[17] Including a cutoff for fever improved predictability (AUC = 0.69). Cattle with low automated lung scores and no fever (<40.3°C) were less likely to die during the feeding period compared with cattle that were only assessed for fever. Based on limited evidence, inclusion of automated lung lesion score could improve BRD prognostic predictions.

Ultrasonography identified significantly more sites with consolidation, pleural irregularities, maximal depth of consolidation, maximal area of consolidation, total consolidated area and affected sites in BRD cattle that died compared with surviving cattle (P-value <.05).[21] However, significant time commitment to perform thorough ultrasonography and adequate training to interpret ultrasonographic images will likely limit the application of ultrasonography in commercial feedlots. More studies are necessary to provide adequate evidence for the effectiveness of both methods.

Treatment outcome prediction based on feedlot records

Feedlots routinely collect valuable treatment and cohort information on individual cattle. Information obtained from various feedlots and several years might be used to predict cattle that will not finish the production cycle (ie, death, culling, premature harvest). Rectal temperature at first BRD diagnosis, days on feed, sex, quarter of the year and body weight on arrival had limited predictive value (area under the curve [AUC] = 0.65) to identify cattle that did not finish the production cycle.[18] Although commonly used, rectal temperature does not seem to predict treatment outcome in feedlot cattle with BRD adequately.

Another study used retrospective treatment records and arrival time (month, quarter, and year) of 23 feedyards collected over 10 years to train, optimize, and evaluate 9 classifiers that identify cattle not finishing the production cycle.[19] Some classification methods had an almost perfect accuracy (95%) on specific subgroups of cattle, but the dataset (feedlot identity) highly influenced the accuracy to detect cattle not finishing the production cycle, which resulted in limited generalizability.[19] Identification of the correct classification method for individual feedlots should be further explored and could enable targeted management of high-risk cattle at the time of first BRD treatment.

IMPLICATIONS AND LIMITATIONS

Results of this systematic review enable veterinarians, researchers, and producers to compare the various methods and technologies currently available to confirm and detect BRD and predict detrimental BRD outcome. Economic considerations of methods to confirm and early detect BRD or prognostic methods should always precede investment in commercial feedlots. One study suggested early detection methods need to cost less than CAD 4.06 per steer to improve economic revenues for commercial feedlots in Canada and the United States.[50] A recent economic analysis additionally reiterated the need for more specific methods, because increasing specificity created more rapid, positive change in net returns compared with increasing sensitivity.[12] The economic values of BRD confirmation, early detection, and prognostic ability differ based on the specific application and current situation; therefore, each feedyard should evaluate the potential cost:benefit ratio of applying improved BRD detection methods in their operation.

By no means can this study claim completeness in all available technologies or methodologies that could be used for improving confirmation, early detection, or prognosis of BRD. Instead, this review summarized the technologies or methodologies that have been applied on feedlot cattle of a certain type (freshly weaned to yearling) and evaluated for effectiveness in BRD detection, confirmation, or prognosis. Technology is evolving quickly and new systems for BRD detection, confirmation, or prognosis are likely. Examples are feeding behavior monitoring systems based on accelerometers,[51] feedbunk antennas detecting tags attached to the leg[52] and alternative location monitoring systems. A remote early disease identification system using location monitoring to track changes in cattle location, activity, and social patterns has been shown to have fair agreement with visual observation for BRD detection.[53] Remote monitoring systems may have an advantage over visual observation owing to the constant monitoring of cattle behavior and the remote early disease identification system illustrated identification of BRD cattle 0.75 days before visual observation. As technology continues to evolve, cattle health care providers will have to determine the optimum ways to incorporate new methodologies to improve BRD diagnostics in a cost-effective manner.

The major limitation of research evaluating diagnosis of BRD is the lack of a gold standard to define a truly BRD-affected animal, which affects the ability to accurately evaluate the sensitivity and specificity of methods or technologies used to detect and diagnose BRD. The true gold standard for BRD can only be a pathologic post mortem evaluation immediately after diagnosis of BRD, which for ethical and economic reasons, is usually avoided. Therefore, every research group developed their own definition of a "true" BRD case. The studies evaluated in this review used clinical illness scoring and rectal temperature cutoffs (between 39.5 and 40.5°C) to verify disease status.

SUMMARY

Numerous methods have been examined to improve BRD diagnosis related to confirmation, early detection, and estimating prognosis. Existing evidence supports the use of HAP to confirm BRD status, but there was limited value for WBC counts and bacteriology in confirming BRD cases. Initial studies using breath analysis, lung ultrasonography, and percutaneous lung biopsy did not provide promising results for BRD confirmation. Early detection of BRD has been successfully performed using IRT, ruminal temperature boluses and feeding behavior monitoring systems. Although promising in infection trials, further studies are necessary to evaluate sensitivities and specificities of location monitoring systems, accelerometers, and pedometers for the use of early BRD detection in naturally occurring BRD. Prognostic methods using routinely collected treatment and cohort data at the time of treatment can be used to identify cattle at risk of unfavorable outcome (ie, cattle dying or not finishing the production cycle).

REFERENCES

1. US Department of Agriculture (USDA). Feedlot 2011 part IV: health and health management on U.S. feedlots with a capacity of 1,000 or more head. Ft Collins (CO): USDA-APIS-VS-CEH-NAHMS; 2013.
2. Cernicchiaro N, White BJ, Renter DG, et al. Evaluation of economic and performance outcomes associated with the number of treatments after an initial diagnosis of bovine respiratory disease in commercial feeder cattle. Am J Vet Res 2013;74:300-9.
3. Schneider MJ, Tait RG, Busby WD, et al. An evaluation of bovine respiratory disease complex in feedlot cattle: impact on performance and carcass traits using treatment records and lung lesion scores. J Anim Sci 2009;87:1821-7.
4. Jim K. Impact of bovine respiratory disease (BRD) from the perspective of the Canadian beef producer. Anim Health Res Rev 2009;10:109-10.
5. Gardner BA, Dolezal HG, Bryant LK, et al. Health of finishing steers: effects on performance, carcass traits, and meat tenderness. J Anim Sci 1999;77:3168-75.
6. White BJ, Renter DG. Bayesian estimation of the performance of using clinical observations and harvest lung lesions for diagnosing bovine respiratory disease in post-weaned beef calves. J Vet Diagn Invest 2009;21:446-53.
7. Weary DM, Huzzey JM, von Keyserlingk MA. Board-invited review: using behavior to predict and identify ill health in animals. J Anim Sci 2009;87:770-7.
8. Timsit E, Bareille N, Seegers H, et al. Visually undetected fever episodes in newly received beef bulls at a fattening operation: occurrence, duration, and impact on performance. J Anim Sci 2011;89:4272-80.
9. Janzen ED, Stockdale PH, Acres SD, et al. Therapeutic and prophylactic effects of some antibiotics on experimental pneumonic pasteurellosis. Can Vet J 1984; 25:78-81.
10. Ferran AA, Toutain PL, Bousquet-Melou A. Impact of early versus later fluoroquinolone treatment on the clinical; microbiological and resistance outcomes in a mouse-lung model of Pasteurella multocida infection. Vet Microbiol 2011;148: 292-7.
11. Griffin D, Chengappa MM, Kuszak J, et al. Bacterial pathogens of the bovine respiratory disease complex. Vet Clin North Am Food Anim Pract 2010;26:381-94.

12. Theurer ME, White BJ, Larson RL, et al. A stochastic model to determine the economic value of changing diagnostic test characteristics for identification of cattle for treatment of bovine respiratory disease. J Anim Sci 2015;93:1398–410.

13. Griffin D. The monster we don't see: subclinical BRD in beef cattle. Anim Health Res Rev 2014;15:138–41.

14. Young I, Waddell L, Sanchez J, et al. The application of knowledge synthesis methods in agri-food public health: recent advancements, challenges and opportunities. Prev Vet Med 2014;113:339–55.

15. Moher D, Liberati A, Tetzlaff J, et al. Preferred reporting items for systematic reviews and meta-analyses: the PRISMA Statement. Open Med 2009;3: e123–30.

16. Deblitz C, Dhuyvetter K. Cost of production and competitiveness of beef production in Canada, the US and the EU. Braunschweig: Thünen Institute of Farm Economics, Working paper 2013/5, English, Available online at: http://www. agribenchmark.org/fileadmin/Dateiablage/B-Beef-and-Sheep/Working-Paper/bs-05-USEU-neu.pdf.

17. Noffsinger T, Brattain K, Quakenbush G, et al. Field results from whisper stethoscope studies. Anim Health Res Rev 2014;15:142–4.

18. Theurer ME, White BJ, Larson RL, et al. Relationship between rectal temperature at first treatment for bovine respiratory disease complex in feedlot calves and the probability of not finishing the production cycle. J Am Vet Med Assoc 2014;245: 1279–85.

19. Amrine DE, White BJ, Larson RL. Comparison of classification algorithms to predict outcomes of feedlot cattle identified and treated for bovine respiratory disease. Comput Electron Agr 2014;105:9–19.

20. Quimby WF, Sowell BF, Bowman JG, et al. Application of feeding behaviour to predict morbidity of newly received calves in a commercial feedlot. Can J Anim Sci 2001;81:315–20.

21. Rademacher RD, Buczinski S, Tripp HM, et al. Systematic thoracic ultrasonography in acute bovine respiratory disease of feedlot steers: impact of lung consolidation on diagnosis and prognosis in a case-control study. Bov Pract 2014;48:1–10.

22. Abutarbush SM, Pollock CM, Wildman BK, et al. Evaluation of the diagnostic and prognostic utility of ultrasonography at first diagnosis of presumptive bovine respiratory disease. Can J Vet Res 2012;76:23–32.

23. Burgess BA, Hendrick SH, Pollock CM, et al. The use of lung biopsy to determine early lung pathology and its association with health and production outcomes in feedlot steers. Can J Vet Res 2013;77:281–7.

24. Idoate I, Vander Ley B, Schultz L, et al. Acute phase proteins in naturally occurring respiratory disease of feedlot cattle. Vet Immunol Immunopathol 2015;163: 221–6.

25. Allen JW, Viel L, Bateman KG, et al. Cytological findings in bronchoalveolar lavage fluid from feedlot calves - associations with pulmonary microbial-flora. Can J Vet Res 1992;56:122–6.

26. Allen JW, Viel L, Bateman KG, et al. The microbial-flora of the respiratory-tract in feedlot calves - associations between nasopharyngeal and bronchoalveolar lavage cultures. Can J Vet Res 1991;55:341–6.

27. Purdy CW, Loan RW, Straus DC, et al. Conglutinin and immunoconglutinin titers in stressed calves in a feedlot. Am J Vet Res 2000;61:1403–9.

28. Timsit E, Assié S, Quiniou R, et al. Early detection of bovine respiratory disease in young bulls using reticulo-rumen temperature boluses. Vet J 2011;190:136–42.

29. Wolfger B, Schwartzkopf-Genswein KS, Barkema HW, et al. Feeding behavior as an early predictor of bovine respiratory disease in North American feedlot systems. J Anim Sci 2015;93:377–85.

30. Buhman MJ, Perino LJ, Galyean ML, et al. Association between changes in eating and drinking behaviors and respiratory tract disease in newly arrived calves at a feedlot. Am J Vet Res 2000;61:1163–8.

31. Sowell BF, Branine ME, Bowman JG, et al. Feeding and watering behavior of healthy and morbid steers in a commercial feedlot. J Anim Sci 1999;77:1105–12.

32. Burciaga-Robles LO, Holland BP, Step DL, et al. Evaluation of breath biomarkers and serum haptoglobin concentration for diagnosis of bovine respiratory disease in heifers newly arrived at a feedlot. Am J Vet Res 2009;70:1291–8.

33. Schaefer AL, Cook NJ, Bench C, et al. The non-invasive and automated detection of bovine respiratory disease onset in receiver calves using infrared thermography. Res Vet Sci 2012;93:928–35.

34. Schaefer AL, Cook NJ, Church JS, et al. The use of infrared thermography as an early indicator of bovine respiratory disease complex in calves. Res Vet Sci 2007; 83:376–84.

35. Buczinski S, Rademacher RD, Tripp HM, et al. Assessment of l-lactatemia as a predictor of respiratory disease recognition and severity in feedlot steers. Prev Vet Med 2014;118:306–18.

36. Berry BA, Krehbiel CR, Confer AW, et al. Effects of dietary energy and starch concentrations for newly received feedlot calves: I. Growth performance and health. J Anim Sci 2004;82:837–44.

37. Taylor JD, Holland BP, Step DL, et al. Nasal isolation of *Mannheimia haemolytica* and *Pasteurella multocida* as predictors of respiratory disease in shipped calves. Res Vet Sci 2015;99:41–5.

38. White BJ, Hanzlicek G, Sanderson MW, et al. Mollicutes species and *Mycoplasma bovis* prevalence and association with health outcomes in beef feeder calves at arrival and initial treatment for bovine respiratory disease. Can Vet J 2010;51:1016–8.

39. Burciaga-Robles LO, Step DL, Krehbiel CR, et al. Effects of exposure to calves persistently infected with bovine viral diarrhea virus type 1b and subsequent infection with *Mannheima haemolytica* on clinical signs and immune variables: model for bovine respiratory disease via viral and bacterial interaction. J Anim Sci 2010;88:2166–78.

40. Aich P, Babiuk LA, Potter AA, et al. Biomarkers for prediction of bovine respiratory disease outcome. OMICS 2009;13:199–209.

41. Rose-Dye TK, Burciaga-Robles LO, Krehbiel CR, et al. Rumen temperature change monitored with remote rumen temperature boluses after challenges with bovine viral diarrhea virus and *Mannheimia haemolytica*. J Anim Sci 2011;89:1193–200.

42. Hanzlicek GA, White BJ, Mosier D, et al. Serial evaluation of physiologic, pathological, and behavioral changes related to disease progression of experimentally induced *Mannheimia haemolytica* pneumonia in postweaned calves. Am J Vet Res 2010;71:359–69.

43. Theurer ME, Anderson DE, White BJ, et al. Effect of *Mannheimia haemolytica* pneumonia on behavior and physiologic responses of calves during high ambient environmental temperatures. J Anim Sci 2013;91:3917–29.

44. McCorkell R, Wynne-Edwards K, Windeyer C, et al. Limited efficacy of Fever Tag temperature sensing ear tags in calves with naturally occurring bovine respiratory disease or induced bovine viral diarrhea virus infection. Can Vet J 2014;55: 688–90.

45. Jones ML, Allison RW. Evaluation of the ruminant complete blood cell count. Vet Clin North Am Food Anim Pract 2007;23:377–402.

46. Salak-Johnson JL, McGlone JJ. Making sense of apparently conflicting data: stress and immunity in swine and cattle. J Anim Sci 2007;85:E81–8.

47. DeVane CL. Substance P: a new era, a new role. Pharmacotherapy 2001;21: 1061–9.

48. Grandin T. Assessment of stress during handling and transport. J Anim Sci 1997; 75:249–57.

49. Hart BL. Biological basis of the behavior of sick animals. Neurosci Biobehav Rev 1988;12:123–37.

50. Wolfger B, Manns BJ, Barkema HW, et al. Evaluating the cost implications of a radio frequency identification feeding system for early detection of bovine respiratory disease in feedlot cattle. Prev Vet Med 2015;118:285–92.

51. Wolfger B, Timsit E, Pajor E, et al. Technical note: accuracy of an ear tag-attached accelerometer to monitor rumination and feeding behavior in feedlot cattle. J Anim Sci 2015. http://dx.doi.org/10.2527/jas2014-8802.

52. Wolfger B, Mang AF, Cook N, et al. Technical note: evaluation of a system for monitoring individual feeding behavior and activity in beef cattle. J Anim Sci, in press. http://dx.doi.org/10.2527/jas2015-894.

53. White BJ, Goehl DR, Amrine DE. Comparison of Remote Early Disease Identification (REDI) system to visual observations to identify cattle with bovine respiratory disease. Int J Appl Res Vet Med 2015;13(1):23–30.

Bovine Viral Diarrhea Virus–Associated Disease in Feedlot Cattle

Robert L. Larson, DVM, PhD, ACT, ACVPM-Epi, ACAN

KEYWORDS

- Bovine viral diarrhea virus • Feedlot cattle • Immunosuppression • Vaccination
- Screening test

KEY POINTS

- Bovine viral diarrhea virus (BVDv) has immunosuppressive and direct effects that interact with other risk factors to impact the likelihood and severity of bovine respiratory disease complex (BRDC) in feedlot cattle.
- Vaccination of feedlot cattle against BVDv antigens is commonly practiced in North American feedlots and a relatively small amount of research data support this intervention as being effective to reduce the likelihood or severity of BRDC.
- Several tests are available to determine if cattle are persistently infected (PI) with BVDv and these tests have high sensitivity and specificity.
- Because of the low prevalence of feedlot cattle PI with BVDv, many positive test results are false-positive.
- Selection of the optimum strategy to use available tests for PI status depends on having an accurate estimate of the cost of PI cattle to feedlot production.

INTRODUCTION

Bovine viral diarrhea virus (BVDv) refers to a heterogeneous group of viruses that belong to 2 different species, BVDv1 and BVDv2, within the pestivirus genus of the Flavivirus family.[1] Bovine viral diarrhea viruses are further subclassified as cytopathic and

Disclosures: During the past 5 years, Dr B.L. Larson has materially participated in research funded through a variety of sources including: Kansas State University Department of Clinical Sciences, the United States Department of Agriculture, the National Cattlemen's Beef Association, Merck Animal Health, Zoetis Animal Health, and CEVA Biomune. He has performed consulting or training activities for: Alpharma Animal Health, Bayer Animal Health, Boehringer-Ingelheim, Elanco Animal Health, IDEXX, Merck Animal Health, Merial, Novartis Animal Health, and Zoetis Animal Health.
Coleman Chair Food Animal Production Medicine, Department of Clinical Sciences, College of Veterinary Medicine, Kansas State University, 111B Mosier Hall, Manhattan, KS 66506, USA
E-mail address: Rlarson@vet.ksu.edu

noncytopathic based on their activity in cultured epithelial cells, with noncytopathic BVDv predominating in nature.[1] These viruses are associated with a number of feedlot cattle diseases; primarily bovine respiratory disease complex (BRDC) and to a lesser frequency, digestive tract disease.

BOVINE VIRAL DIARRHEA VIRUS AND BOVINE RESPIRATORY DISEASE COMPLEX

BRDC is an important disease of cattle and is causally associated with a number of identified and suspected risk factors, including infection with BVDv.[2–4] Although, BVDv alone (uncomplicated by co-infection or serial-infection with other agents) has been demonstrated to cause respiratory infection and signs of clinical BRDC in experimental challenge studies,[5–7] reviews of numerous studies have concluded that BVDv association with BRDC is most importantly due to suppression of the immune system and synergism with other pathogens.[8–10]

IMMUNOSUPPRESSION ASSOCIATED WITH BOVINE VIRAL DIARRHEA VIRUS INFECTION

Brakenbury and colleagues,[7] summarized evidence that infection with BVDv results in immunosuppression in the absence of clinical signs of primary BVDv-induced disease. Experimental studies found that acute infections with BVDv enhanced susceptibility to infection with bovine herpes virus 1,[11] and case reports have linked concurrent infections with other BRDC-associated pathogens with BVDv infections.[12] Subsequent experimental studies showed healthy cattle exposed to BVDv responded differently to a challenge with *Mannheimia haemolytica* than calves not previously exposed to BVDv.[13]

Ridpath[8] reviewed available literature and concluded that the immunosuppression that accompanies acute BVDv infections results from a combination of outright lymphoid cell death[14,15] and reduced function in remaining lymphoid cells.[10] Although the mechanism remains undefined, infection with either high- or low-virulence BVDv results in the reduction of circulating lymphocytes[14–16] and the depletion of lymphoid tissue.[17,18] The difference in pathology between high-virulence and low-virulence BVDv strains is in the extent of cell death or loss, with reduction of circulating lymphocytes and lymphoid depletion being significantly higher after infection with highly virulent BVDv.[8]

Peterhans and colleagues[9] and Chase and colleagues[10] summarized the literature relating to the immune response to BVDv and reported that in addition to reducing lymphoid cell numbers, BVDv infections impair the function of cells associated with both the acquired and innate immune systems. The interactions resulting in immune suppression are complex and components of the innate immune response that are reported to be suppressed in response to BVDv infection include interferon production, phagocytosis, chemotaxis, and microbiocidal killing. On the acquired immune side, changes such as downregulation of major histocompatibility complex II and interleukin-2 that suppress T-helper cell response and apoptosis of T and B cells in lymphoid tissue are critical immunosuppressive mechanisms.[10]

PERSISTENTLY INFECTED CATTLE AS THE MOST IMPORTANT RESERVOIR FOR BOVINE VIRAL DIARRHEA VIRUS
Creation of Cattle Persistently Infected with Bovine Viral Diarrhea Virus

Several pathogens associated with important diseases of cattle are able to establish a persistently infected (PI) state, but the method by which BVDv creates a PI state is unique. Rather than evading the adaptive immune response of an immune-competent animal, noncytopathic BVDv is able to establish PI by invading the fetus early in its intrauterine development, before the development of a competent immune response, thus establishing immunotolerance that is specific for the persisting viral strain.[9]

Even mild or subclinical infections of susceptible breeding females can cause conception failure, early embryonic loss, abortion, or vertical fetal infection. Fetal infection can lead to early embryonic death, abortion, congenital defects, the birth of PI calves, or the birth of normal calves. The immune status of the dam, the stage of gestation at the time of infection, and the viral biotype are important factors in determining the result of vertical infection. Transplacental infection occurs with high efficiency of seronegative dams[19,20]; however, naturally acquired immunity is considered to provide good, but not necessarily complete, protection against fetal infection.[21] Fetal infection early in the gestation of susceptible dams with a cytopathic biotype of BVDv will result in abortion. However, fetal infection before the development of immune competence with a noncytopathic biotype of BVDv will result either in abortion, or in a certain percentage of infections, the survival of a calf that is immunotolerant to and PI with that noncytopathic strain of BVDv.[20,22] Age at immune competence in the face of BVDv exposure is variable and has been reported to range from 90 to 125 days.[20,22,23] If PI fetuses survive to term, they are continually infected, but immunotolerant to the homologous BVDv.[23,24]

Role of Cattle Persistently Infected with Bovine Viral Diarrhea Virus as Viral Reservoir

Cattle PI with BVDv are the primary reservoir for the virus, with transiently infected cattle considered a less important source. PI animals are more efficient transmitters of BVDv than transiently infected animals because they secrete much higher levels of virus for a much longer period of time. In experimentally challenged, transiently infected cattle, the median minimum number of days until BVDv shedding was detected was 2 days.[25] The median peak of BVDv shedding occurred at 7 days after challenge with shedding ending at a median of 12 days after challenge.[25] In contrast, PI animals usually have a very high and persistent viremia,[26] and BVDv is shed throughout life from virtually all secretions and excretions, including nasal discharge, saliva, semen, urine, tears, milk, and to a lesser extent, feces.[27–29] Horizontal transmission of BVDv to seronegative cattle has been shown to occur after only 1 hour of direct contact with a single PI animal.[30]

Transiently infected cattle are considered to be far less efficient at transmitting BVDv to susceptible animals than PI cattle.[31,32] However, seroconversion among assembled cattle without the presence of PI animals indicates that transmission from transiently infected animals does occur, although spread is considered to be slower.[33,34]

Although mortality of PI calves before weaning has been reported to be very high due to fatal congenital defects and secondary infections that cause enteritis, pneumonia, and arthritis,[35,36] an important percentage survive to weaning and studies have reported 0.2% to 0.4% of cattle entering US feedlots to be PI with BVDv.[4,37–39]

Direct Health Risk of Bovine Viral Diarrhea Virus Persistently Infected Feedlot Cattle

In a study that evaluated lung pathology and infectious agents associated with deaths in a single feedyard over a 1-year period, 0.70% of cattle in the study died of BRDC and 5.3% of cattle that died due to BRDC were estimated to be BVDv PI.[40] Assuming that the percentage of BVDv PI cattle arriving at the feedlot was similar to that reported in other studies (ie, 0.2%–0.4%), BVDv PI cattle are much more likely to die due to BRDC than non-PI cattle. The negative effect on mortality risk of feedlot cattle being

BVDv PI was also reported in a study in which 25.6% of cattle PI for BVDv at feedlot arrival died compared with 2.4% of non-PI cattle.[41] An earlier study also showed that BVDv PI cattle were more common in populations of dead cattle (2.5%) and chronically ill cattle (2.6%) than in cattle arriving at a feedyard (0.3%).[4]

The US Department of Agriculture estimates 23.8 million cattle were placed on feed in the United States in 2011 and 2.0% of cattle (476,000 head) placed on feed died or were sent to market before reaching desired slaughter weight.[42] Estimates from published research indicate that 0.2% to 0.4% (47,600–95,200) of cattle arriving at US feedlots are PI for BVDv[4,37–39] and 25.6% of PI cattle (12,000–24,400) die before slaughter,[41] meaning that eliminating BVDv PIs from the US beef population would decrease feedlot losses by approximately 12,000 to 24,400 animals per year (ie, decrease losses from 2% of placements to 1.90%–1.95% of placements) due to direct effects of losses of BVDv PI cattle. Therefore, although direct losses due to BVDv PI cattle in the feedlot are measureable, addressing other contributions to feedlot losses probably takes priority.

Health Risk of Feedlot Cattle in Contact with Bovine Viral Diarrhea Virus Persistently Infected Cattle

In addition to the direct losses of cattle PI with BVDv, feedlots may experience losses among non-PI cattle that are transiently infected with BVDv due to transmission of the virus from PI cattle. Transmission of BVDv from PI cattle to in-contact susceptible cattle occurs during marketing, trucking, and while in feeding pens and pastures.[43] The likelihood and extent of health and growth performance effects of non-PI feedlot cattle being exposed to BVDv PI cattle has been reported to vary greatly, including both positive and negative effects. BVDv viremia or seroconversion has been associated with respiratory disease outbreaks in feedlot situations.[2–4] Loneragan and colleagues[4] reported that exposure to a PI animal appeared to have little effect when exposure was narrowly defined to include just those cattle within the pen of a PI animal. However, when exposure was defined more broadly to include pens adjacent to a pen containing a PI animal, exposure had a detectable adverse effect on risk of illness compared with not-exposed cattle. The risk of initial treatment for respiratory tract disease was 43% (95% confidence interval [CI] 2%–102%) greater in cattle exposed to a PI animal in the same or adjacent pen, compared with those not exposed to a PI animal. Overall, 15.9% of initial respiratory tract disease events were attributable to exposure to a PI animal.[4]

Similarly, Hessman and colleagues[41] not only evaluated the risk of cattle in the same feedlot pen as cattle PI for BVDv throughout the feeding phase, but also cattle in pens adjacent to pens containing PI cattle throughout the feeding phase, as well as cattle that were in the same pen or next to pens with PI cattle that were identified and removed within 72 hours of feedlot arrival. The investigators found that pens of cattle that did not have any PI cattle at the time of feedlot arrival and adjacent pens also lacked PI cattle or PI cattle were removed within 72 hours had significantly higher weight gain than pens with PI cattle present at arrival, whether or not those PI cattle were removed within 72 hours.[41] The same study found that cattle in feedlot pens with PI cattle present either in the same pen throughout the feeding phase or present for 72 hours or less (PI cattle in the pen were removed within 72 hours) and exposed to PI cattle in adjacent pens throughout feeding, were more likely to be identified as ill than cattle in pens with no PI cattle at arrival and PI cattle in adjacent pens were removed within 72 hours.[41]

However, exposure to BVDv PI cattle or seroconversion to BVDv after feedlot entry is not always reported to have a negative association. In a study investigating the risk factors of commingling and presence of PI cattle in feedlot pens, disease prevalence (mean ± SD morbidity, 7.9% ± 3.1%) was lowest in pens containing single-source cattle and a BVDv PI calf; and in pens with commingled cattle, the presence of a PI animal (mean morbidity 28.6% ± 10.1%) was not associated with increased disease prevalence compared with pens without PI cattle (mean morbidity, 29.3% ± 16.22%)[38] A study that used polymerase chain reaction (PCR) analysis of blood samples collected at feedlot arrival to identify initial BVDv infection status and immunohistochemistry of a skin biopsy to identify BVDv PI status found that presence of PI cattle did not have a large negative impact on pen-level health and growth performance outcomes in feedlot cattle.[44]

A study that evaluated the effect of either short-term (ie, 60 hours) or long-term (throughout feeding phase) exposure of BVDv-vaccinated feedlot heifers to PI cattle did not identify a negative effect of either exposure length on health, growth performance, or carcass characteristics compared with unexposed controls.[45] Even in the study reported by Hessman and colleagues,[41] pens of cattle with the least exposure to PI cattle (ie, no PI at arrival and no exposure to PI cattle at any time during feeding) did not have the lowest morbidity percentage, first relapse percentage, fatality percentage, treatment costs, or mean number of treatments per illness compared with pens with some exposure to PI cattle. Based on currently available studies, the direction and magnitude of response of feedlot cattle exposed to BVDv PI cattle cannot be predicted. A number of reviews have suggested that the range in response of feedlot cattle to BVDv exposure could be due to variation in virulence or pathogenicity characteristics of specific BVDv to which cattle are exposed; immune status of the exposed cattle; extent of concurrent or serial exposure to other infectious, physiologic, or metabolic insults; or other unknown risk factors.[8,46–48]

CONSIDERATIONS OF BOVINE VIRAL DIARRHEA VIRUS SPECIES AND STRAINS (SUBTYPES)

Studies have indicated that US feedlot cattle are infected with diverse species of BVDv. Fulton and colleagues[49] reported that using accessions to an Oklahoma diagnostic laboratory representing clinically ill or necropsied cattle during the year 2005, that 45.8% of isolates were BVDv-1b, whereas 28.2% were BVDv-1a, and 26.0% were BVDv-2a. Similarly, a study of isolates from PI cattle in southwestern US feedlots reported that 75.3% were BVDv-1b, 12.6% were BVDv-2a, and 12.1% were BVDv-1a.[50]

Some studies have shown differences in responses between strains in in vitro studies. Walz and colleagues[51] found that in colostrum-deprived Holstein calves, altered platelet function was observed in calves infected with 2 type II BVDv isolates (BVDv 890 and BVDv 7937), but was not observed in calves infected with a type I BVDv (BVDv TGAN). The same research group also reported that pathologic and immunohistochemical examinations revealed more pronounced lesions and more extensive distribution of viral antigen in colostrum-deprived calves inoculated with 2 type II BVDv (BVDv 890 and BVDv 7937) compared with calves inoculated with a type I BVDv (BVDv TGAN).[52]

Other studies have demonstrated differences at the animal level or pen level between cattle that seroconvert to different species of BVDv. Booker and colleagues[44] reported that cattle that were in pens that contained animals with type I BVDv infections had significantly more initial BRDC treatments, and overall mortalities, than cattle in pens that did not include PI cattle. In addition, individual cattle that seroconverted to BVDv type I infection were approximately 4 times more likely to die of all causes than to animals without BVDv type I infection. Moreover, at the pen level, seroconverting to BVDv type II appeared to convey a protective effect when compared with pens without BVDv type II infections.[44] Although there is some evidence for different outcomes based on exposure to different BVDv species, it is not clear that outcome severity can be directly related to species differences between BVDv-1 and BVDv-2.

BOVINE VIRAL DIARRHEA VIRUS ASSOCIATION WITH DISEASES OTHER THAN BOVINE RESPIRATORY DISEASE COMPLEX IN FEEDLOT CATTLE

Although very little published literature exists to document the extent and characteristics of non-BRDC, BVDv-associated disease in North American feedlots, some case reports and anecdotal information suggest a potential sporadic association of BVDv with severe digestive tract disease.[53–55] Hessman and colleagues[55] report a case of BVDv infection in non-PI feedlot cattle in 2 arrival cohorts in a single feedlot causing severe mucosal surface lesions in the oral cavity, larynx, and esophagus. The cumulative morbidity and mortality losses were 76.2% and 30.8%, respectively, for one cohort and 49.0% and 5.6% respectively for the other cohort.[55] Other evidence of association between BVDv and digestive tract pathology is reported in experimental challenge of young, seronegative calves,[56–58] which may not have direct relevance to cattle in typical feedlot settings.

ROLE OF VACCINATION IN THE MANAGEMENT OF BOVINE VIRAL DIARRHEA VIRUS IN FEEDLOT SETTINGS

Vaccination against BVDv antigens at the time cattle arrive at a feedlot as well as earlier in the cattle production system is a common intervention to reduce the biologic and economic costs of BVDv in feedlot cattle.[42,59] Terrell and colleagues[59] surveyed feedlot veterinarians providing cattle health and well-being recommendations for feedlot cattle in the United States and Canada and found that all surveyed veterinarians recommended that high-risk cattle be vaccinated with BVDv (types 1 and 2) vaccine, and 95.65% recommended that low-risk cattle be vaccinated with BVDv (types 1 and 2) vaccine. However, very little clinical trial data exist illustrating the efficacy of vaccination at feedlot arrival to prevent BVDv infection and clinical disease associated with BVDv.

Three days before exposure to cattle PI with BVDv-1b, Fulton and colleagues,[60] vaccinated cattle with a modified live viral (MLV) vaccine containing BVDv-1a and BVDv-2a and found that BVDv-1b was transmitted to both vaccinated cattle and unvaccinated controls. For cattle that were vaccinated at the ranch of origin and were seropositive for BVDv before PI exposure, BVDv-1b titers up to 64 did not prevent BVDv-1b from being isolated after exposure. In fact, BVDv-1b antibody titers up to 256 did not uniformly prevent fourfold or greater rises in BVDv-1b antibody titers. The investigators concluded that even though the vaccinated calves responded with antibodies against BVDv, the onset of immunity preventing infection to a heterologous BVDv-1b strain requires more than 3 days.[60] Grooms and colleagues[48] reported a series of trials and found in one trial that cattle vaccinated against BVDv within 24 hours of feedlot arrival had lower morbidity risk than unvaccinated cattle when the cattle were exposed to PI cattle; however, in an another study, they did not detect a difference in health and growth performance after exposure to PI cattle depending on whether cattle were or were not vaccinated against BVDv.

Theurer and colleagues[61] did a systematic review and meta-analysis of the effectiveness of commercially available vaccines against BVDv and other viral pathogens associated with BRDC. They identified only 2 field studies that reported the effects of 5 trials that compared cattle vaccinated against BVDv, bovine herpes virus-1 (infectious bovine rhinotracheitis), bovine respiratory syncytial virus, and parinfluenza-3 virus with unvaccinated controls on mortality and/or morbidity risk.[62,63] Randomized controlled blinded field trials in commercial feedlots provide assurance of high internal study validity due to their ability to control for common sources of bias and confounding, and a high level of external validity for veterinarians advising feedlot managers, as the host, environment, and pathogen triad are expected to be similar to typical feedlot production settings. Analysis of these 5 trials revealed a significantly lower morbidity risk for vaccinates compared with controls in 2 of the 5 trials, with no significant difference between groups in the remaining 3 trials.[61] The summary morbidity risk ratio for these 5 trials was 0.44 with a 95% CI of 0.26–0.74; this is interpreted as "Vaccination against the viruses included in the studied commercially available vaccines is estimated to decrease morbidity risk by about 44% with potential true reduction ranging from 26% to 74%, which is a significantly lower morbidity risk for vaccinated beef calves compared with that for non-vaccinated control calves."[61] Therefore, if the group of cattle was going to have 30% morbidity without vaccination, they would be expected to have between 8% and 22% morbidity, with the most likely estimate of 17% if they were vaccinated. Mortality risk was reported for only 4 of the trials, and the summarized risk ratio for these 4 trials was 0.19, with a 95% CI of 0.06–0.67; indicating vaccination is expected to reduce mortality risk associated with viruses associated with BRDC by approximately 19% with a true magnitude of effect most likely being somewhere between a 6% to 67% reduced mortality risk for vaccinates, compared with controls.[61]

Although randomized controlled blinded field trials provide a higher level of evidence compared with challenge studies, challenge studies do allow more in-depth evaluation of the pathophysiology of BRDC and the mechanisms of action of protective immunity. However, demonstration of vaccine efficacy in a challenge study does not provide sufficient evidence for similar protection in a clinical setting; therefore, extrapolation of results from disease challenge studies to commercial field settings must be performed with caution. Reviewing challenge studies, Theurer and colleagues[61] identified 7 studies containing 11 trials that evaluated the effectiveness of an MLV BVDv vaccine against experimental infection with BVDv and signs attributable to BRDC in beef or dairy calves. Analysis revealed a significantly lower morbidity risk for vaccinates, compared with controls, in 6 of the 11 trials, with no significant difference between groups in the remaining 5 trials. The summarized risk ratio for these 11 trials was 0.28, with a 95% CI of 0.17–0.45.[61] Two studies comprising 4 trials provided mortality data for MLV vaccinated and nonvaccinated calves after experimental BVDv challenge. The summarized risk ratio for these 4 trials was 0.26, with a 95% CI of 0.12–0.56, indicating a significantly lower mortality risk for vaccinates than for control calves.[61] Theurer and colleagues[61] also identified 2 studies comprising 2 trials that evaluated the effectiveness of inactivated (killed) BVDv vaccine against infection with BVDv to mitigate signs attributable to BRDC in beef or dairy calves after experimental challenge with the virus. The summarized risk ratio for these 2 trials was 0.66, but was not significant because of a wide 95% CI of 0.35–1.26 for morbidity risk between vaccinates and control calves. One study comprising 2 trials evaluated mortality risk for calves that did or did not receive inactivated BVDv vaccine before BVDv challenge. The summarized risk ratio for these 2 trials was 0.12, with a 95% CI of 0.02–0.79, indicating a significantly lower mortality risk for vaccinates than for control calves.[61]

Theurer and colleagues[61] conclude that although the available data support the use of vaccines directed against BVDv in feedlot cattle, published natural challenge field studies with blinded evaluation of clinically important outcomes are sparse. In addition, extrapolation of positive challenge study evaluations of BVDv vaccine effectiveness in controlled settings to field settings is not wholly appropriate. More research needs to be published based on studies done in field settings with natural exposure to evaluate currently available vaccine effectiveness as measured by clinically relevant outcomes with adequate blinding of evaluators to treatment groups and appropriate study design to truly determine the magnitude and direction of vaccine efficacy, as Perino and Hunsaker[64] previously described.

ROLE OF TESTING AND REMOVAL OF PERSISTENTLY INFECTED CATTLE IN THE MANAGEMENT OF BOVINE VIRAL DIARRHEA VIRUS IN FEEDLOT SETTINGS

The unique method by which BVDv establishes a PI state in the in utero fetus provides an opportunity to test for PI status at any time in an animal's life with the confidence that an accurate PI-status determination will remain the same throughout life. In other words, cattle that are truly negative for BVDv PI status cannot become PI at a later time point, and cattle truly positive for BVDv PI status cannot clear the infection and become PI-negative. Because of this constant PI status and the understanding that a small percentage of cattle are PI with BVDv and constitute the primary reservoir for the virus, testing and removal of PI cattle at feedlot arrival or earlier can effectively remove nearly all the BVDv reservoir from the population if the test returns few false-negative results.

A number of diagnostic tests with good accuracy to identify BVDv PI status are available. Nickell and colleagues[65] reviewed the published estimates for sensitivity and specificity of available BVDv PI tests and reported that:

- Immunohistochemistry is expected to have a sensitivity of 99.6% (minimum 97.6% and maximum 100.0%) and a specificity of 99.6% (minimum 98.8% and maximum 100%)
- Antigen capture enzyme-linked immunosorbent assay is expected to have a sensitivity of 100% (minimum 98% and maximum 100%) and a specificity of 99.3% (minimum 97.7% and maximum 100%)
- Real-time PCR is expected to have a sensitivity of 100% (minimum 99% and maximum 100%) and a specificity of 100% (minimum 99% and maximum 100%)

Because the sensitivity for each of the available tests is high ($\geq$97.6%) and the prevalence of BVDv PI cattle is low (0.2%–0.4%), nearly all (>99.5%) feedlot cattle if tested at arrival will have a negative test result, and the certainty that a test-negative animal is truly not PI is very high. Using the minimum likely sensitivity of 97.6% and the high end of the expected PI prevalence range of 0.4%, the negative predictive value of BVDv PI tests in US feedlot cattle populations is approximately 99.99%; therefore, at worst, one would expect 1 false-negative test result for every 11,000 tests performed.

In contrast, even though specificity is high for the available tests, because the prevalence of PI cattle at feedlot arrival is low (0.2%–0.4%) and relatively few cattle will test positive for PI status (<0.5%), the certainty that a test-positive animal is truly positive is problematic. Using the minimum likely specificity of 97.7% and the low end of the expected PI prevalence range of 0.2%, the positive predictive value of BVDv PI tests in US feedlot cattle populations could be as poor as approximately 7.84%. Using a specificity of 99.9% and a PI prevalence of 0.4% results in a best-case positive predictive value of 79.7%. In other words, at best, 8 of every 10 positive animals are truly BVDv PI and at worst, fewer than 1 out of every 10 positive animals is truly BVDv PI.

Because the costs associated with euthanizing cattle that have a false-positive BVDv PI test result are high, implementing PI testing in US feedlot populations may require either a 2-test strategy whereby cattle that test positive on an initial test for PI status are retested with a second PI test (with the results of the second test considered to be definitive) to better differentiate between true-positive and false-positive cattle, or to isolate all cattle that test positive on a single PI test (both true-positive and false-positive) away from the rest of the feedlot population to achieve removal of the BVDv reservoir.[37] A negative aspect of the strategy to test for BVDv PI status at feedlot arrival followed by removal of test-positive cattle is the time delay between initial sample collection and identification of PI animals for removal from the population. During this delay, PI cattle would be contacting pen mates and cattle in adjacent pens and potentially causing negative biologic and economic effects. Depending on how test-positive cattle are managed after the initial test, this delay could be increased with a 2-step strategy versus a 1-step testing strategy.

Before widespread adoption of any testing strategy can be recommended, more confidence in the estimated economic return for testing at feedlot arrival is needed, and the relative value of testing at feedlot arrival versus the value to the feedlot phase of production for testing at the ranch of origin or the point of sale (and hence, the price-premium that could be paid) needs to be determined. The economic return of testing for BVDv PI cattle at feedlot arrival will depend on the prevalence of PI cattle, the confidence in results of the testing strategy, the true economic cost of the presence of PI cattle in feedlot operations, and the value of removal of PI cattle after test results are known.

The number of false-positive test results and the cost of testing populations that are not likely to contain PI cattle can be decreased by only testing populations of cattle at feedlot arrival that are considered to be high risk for including PI animals rather than testing all arriving cattle lots. However, this strategy would require that populations that are truly low risk and high risk for including PI cattle can be accurately identified and the strategy would likely result in some PI cattle entering the feedlot in untested (presumed low-risk) populations.

Even though cattle that are identified as BVDv PI at feedlot arrival are much less likely to survive to slaughter weight than other cattle in the feedlot, the health and performance of cattle that actually have false-positive test results are not expected to compare negatively with other non-PI cattle and some true-positive PI cattle will reach a weight that can be economically harvested. Therefore, a strategy to capture value from cattle that test positive for PI status is an important consideration in the economic evaluation of testing. However, any strategy to capture some of the value of PI-test-positive cattle should try to avoid the sale of test-positive animals, or if PI-test-positive cattle are sold, full disclosure to and understanding by the buyer should be ensured. The Academy of Veterinary Consultants, the American Association of Bovine Practitioners, and the National Cattlemen's Beef Association have all developed position statements that acknowledge that appropriate disposition of known PI cattle must take into account the adverse impact those cattle have on the health, welfare, and economic return of the other cattle or cattle operations they may expose to BVDv.[66–68] The statements recognize that cattle PI with BVDv are defective and once confirmed, their PI status should thereafter be disclosed.

SUMMARY

BVDv is associated with BRDC and other diseases of feedlot cattle. Although occasionally a primary pathogen, BVDv's impact on cattle health is most importantly through the immunosuppressive effects of the virus and its synergism with other pathogens. Because BVDv is only one of many risk factors that interact with other pathogens and numerous metabolic, immunologic, and physiologic factors to contribute to disease syndromes of feedlot cattle, the simple presence or absence of the virus does not result in consistent health outcomes. Current interventions available to veterinarians providing services to feedlot operations to address BVDv involve vaccination at feedlot arrival or earlier in beef cattle production, the use of testing for PI status and either euthanasia or segregation of test-positive animals to remove this important BVDv reservoir, and other animal husbandry and health interactions to limit concurrent or serial disease risk factors. All of these interventions have limitations and the optimum strategy for their uses to limit the health, production, and economic costs associated with BVDv have to be carefully considered for optimum cost-effectiveness.

REFERENCES

1. Ridpath JF. Bovine viral diarrhea virus. In: Mahy BW, Regenmortel MH, editors. Encyclopedia of virology. Oxford (United Kingdom): Elsevier; 2008. p. 374–80.
2. Fulton RW, Purdy CW, Confer AW, et al. Bovine viral diarrhea viral infections in feeder calves with respiratory disease: interactions with *Pasteurella* spp., parainfluencza-2 virus, and bovine respiratory syncytial virus. Can J Vet Res 2000;64:151–9.
3. Fulton RW, Ridpath JF, Saliki JT, et al. Bovine viral diarrhea virus (BVDV) 1b: predominant BVDV subtype in calves with respiratory disease. Can J Vet Res 2002; 66:181–90.
4. Loneragan GH, Thomson DU, Montgomery DL, et al. Prevalence, outcome, and health consequences associated with bovine viral diarrhea virus in feedlot cattle. J Am Vet Med Assoc 2005;226:595–601.
5. Potgeiter LN, McCracken MD, Hopkins FM, et al. Experimental production of respiratory tract disease with bovine viral diarrhea virus. Am J Vet Res 1984;45:1582–5.
6. Potgeiter LN, McCracken MD, Hopkins FM, et al. Comparison of pneumopathogencity of two strains of bovine viral diarrhea virus. Am J Vet Res 1985;46:151–3.
7. Brakenbury LS, Carr BV, Charleston B. Aspects of the innate and adaptive immune responses to acute infections with BVDV. Vet Microbiol 2003;96:337–44.
8. Ridpath JF. The contribution of infections with bovine viral diarrhea viruses to bovine respiratory disease. Vet Clin North Am Food Anim Pract 2010;26:335–48.
9. Peterhans E, Jungi TW, Schweizer M. BVD virus and innate immunity. Biologicals 2003;31:107–12.
10. Chase CC, Elmowalid G, Yousif AA. The immune response to bovine viral diarrhea virus: a constantly changing picture. Vet Clin North Am Food Anim Pract 2004;20(1):95–114.
11. Edwards S, Wood L, Hewitt-Taylor C, et al. Evidence for an immunocompromising effect of bovine pestivirus on bovid herpesvirus 1 vaccination. Vet Res Commun 1986;10:297–302.
12. Wray C, Roeder PL. Effect of bovine virus diarrhoea-mucosal disease virus infection on salmonella infection in calves. Res Vet Sci 1987;42:213–8.
13. Burciaga-Robles LO, Step DL, Krehbiel CR, et al. Effects of exposure to calves persistently infected with bovine viral diarrhea virus type 1b and subsequent infection with *Mannheimia haemolytica* on clinical signs and immune variables: model for bovine respiratory disease via viral and bacterial interaction. J Anim Sci 2010;88:2166–78.
14. Ridpath JF, Neill JD, Frey M, et al. Phylogenetic, antigenic and clinical characterization of type 2 BVDV from North America. Vet Microbiol 2000;77(1–2):145–55.

15. Ridpath JF, Neill JD, Peterhans E. Impact of variation in acute virulence of BVDV1 strains on design of better vaccine efficacy challenge models. Vaccine 2007; 25(47):8058–66.

16. Bolin SR, Ridpath JF. Differences in virulence between two noncytopathic bovine viral diarrhea viruses in calves. Am J Vet Res 1992;53(11):2157–63.

17. Liebler-Tenorio EM, Ridpath JE, Neill JD. Distribution of viral antigen and development of lesions after experimental infection with highly virulent bovine viral diarrhea virus type 2 in calves. Am J Vet Res 2002;63(11):1575–84.

18. Liebler-Tenorio EM, Ridpath JF, Neill JD. Distribution of viral antigen and development of lesions after experimental infection of calves with a BVDV 2 strain of low virulence. J Vet Diagn Invest 2003;15(3):221–32.

19. Done JT, Terlecki S, Richardson C, et al. Bovine virus diarrhea-mucosal disease virus: pathogenicity for the fetal calf following maternal infection. Vet Rec 1980; 106:473–9.

20. McClurkin AW, Littledike ET, Cutlip RC, et al. Production of cattle immunotolerant to bovine viral diarrhea virus. Can J Comp Med 1984;48:156–61.

21. Orban S, Liess B, Hafez SM, et al. Studies on transplacental transmissibility of a bovine virus diarrhoea (BVD) vaccine virus. I. Inoculation of pregnant cows 15 to 90 days before parturition (190th to 265th day of gestation). Zentralbl Veterinarmed B 1983;30:619–34.

22. Casaro AP, Kendrick JW, Kennedy PC. Response of the bovine fetus to bovine viral diarrhea-mucosal disease virus. Am J Vet Res 1971;32:1543–62.

23. Roeder PL, Jeffrey M, Cranwell MP. Pestivirus fetopathogenicity in cattle: changing sequelae with fetal maturation. Vet Rec 1986;118:44–8.

24. Duffell SJ, Harkness JW. Bovine virus diarrhea—mucosal disease infection in cattle. Vet Rec 1985;117:240–5.

25. Grissett G, White BJ, Larson RL. Structured literature review of responses of cattle to viral and bacterial pathogens causing bovine respiratory disease complex. J Vet Intern Med 2015;29:770–80.

26. Nickell JS, White BJ, Larson RL, et al. Evidence of viral transmission and nasal excretion of virus without detectable serum viremia among beef calves exposed to a calf persistently infected with bovine viral diarrhea virus. Int J Appl Res Vet Med 2010;8:29–39.

27. Rae AG, Sinclair JA, Nettleton PF. Survival of bovine virus diarrhoea virus in blood from persistently infected cattle. Vet Rec 1987;120:504.

28. Bezek DM, Stofregen D, Posso M. Effect of cytopathic bovine viral diarrhea virus (BVDV) superinfection on viral antigen association with platelets, viremia, and specific antibody levels in two heifers persistently infected with BVDV. J Vet Diagn Invest 1995;7:395–7.

29. Brock KV, Grooms DL, Ridpath J, et al. Changes in levels of viremia in cattle persistently infected with bovine viral diarrhea virus. J Vet Diagn Invest 1998;10:22–6.

30. Traven M, Alenius S, Fossum C, et al. Primary bovine viral diarrhoea virus infection in calves following direct contact with a persistently viraemic calf. Zentralbl Veterinarmed B 1991;38:453–62.

31. Niskanen R, Lindberg A, Larsson B, et al. Lack of virus transmission from bovine viral diarrhoea virus infected calves to susceptible peers. Acta Vet Scand 2000;41:93–9.

32. Niskanen R, Lindberg A, Traven M. Failure to spread bovine virus diarrhoea virus infection from primarily infected calves despite concurrent infection with bovine coronavirus. Vet J 2002;163:251–9.

33. Meyling A, Houe H, Jensen AM. Epidemiology of bovine virus diarrhoea virus. Rev Sci Tech 1990;9:75–93.

34. Moerman A, Straver PJ, de Jong MC, et al. A long term epidemiological study of bovine viral diarrhoea infections in a large herd of dairy cattle. Vet Rec 1993;132: 622–6.
35. Houe H. Survivorship of animals persistently infected with bovine virus diarrhoea virus (BVDV). Prev Vet Med 1993;15:275–83.
36. Graham DA, Clegg TA, O'Sullivan PO, et al. Survival time of calves with positive BVD virus results born during the voluntary phase of the Irish eradication programme. Prev Vet Med 2015;119:123–33. Available at: http://ac.els-cdn.com/S0167587715000653/1-s2.0-S0167587715000653-main.pdf?_tid=0ec94244-d33d-11e4-bdea-00000aab0f27&acdnat=1427322172_edcd37ebb49caadd4897bd1da3631c04.
37. Larson RL, Miller RB, Kleiboeker SB, et al. Economic costs associated with two testing strategies for screening feeder calves for persistent infection with bovine viral diarrhea virus. J Am Vet Med Assoc 2005;226:249–54.
38. O'Connor A, Sorden SD, Apley MD. Association between the existence of calves persistently infected with bovine viral diarrhea virus and commingling on pen morbidity in feedlot cattle. Am J Vet Res 2005;66:2130–4.
39. Fulton RW, Hessman B, Johnson BJ, et al. Evaluation of diagnostic tests used for detection of bovine viral diarrhea virus and prevalence of subtypes 1a, 1b, and 2a in persistently infected cattle entering a feedlot. J Am Vet Med Assoc 2006; 228:578–84.
40. Fulton RW, Blood KS, Panciera RJ, et al. Lung pathology and infectious agents in fatal feedlot pneumonias and relationship with mortality, disease onset, and treatments. J Vet Diagn Invest 2009;21:464–77.
41. Hessman BE, Fulton RW, Sjeklocha DB, et al. Evaluation of economic effects and the health and performance of the general cattle population after exposure to cattle persistently infected with bovine viral diarrhea virus in a starter feedlot. Am J Vet Res 2009;70:73–85.
42. USDA: APHIS:VS: NAHMS Feedlot 2011. Part III: Trends in Health and Management Practices on U.S. Feedlots, 1994-2011. Available at: http://www.aphis.usda.gov/animal_health/nahms/feedlot/downloads/feedlot2011/Feed11_dr_Part%20III.pdf. Accessed January 26, 2015.
43. Grooms DL, Brock KV, Norby B. Performance of feedlot cattle exposed to animals persistently infected with bovine viral diarrhea virus. Proceedings of the 83rd Annual Meeting of the Conference of Research Workers in Animal Diseases. St. Louis (MO), November 11, 2002. [Abstract: #186].
44. Booker CW, Abutarbush SM, Morley PS, et al. The effect of bovine viral diarrhea virus infections on health and performance of feedlot cattle. Can Vet J 2008;49: 253–60.
45. Elam NA, Thomson DU, Gleghorn JF. Effects of long- or short-term exposure to a calf identified as persistently infected with bovine viral diarrhea virus on feedlot performance of freshly weaned, transport-stressed beef heifers. J Anim Sci 2008;86:1917–24.
46. Campbell JR. Effect of bovine viral diarrhea virus in the feedlot. Vet Clin North Am Food Anim Pract 2004;20:39–50.
47. Ridpath JF, Fulton RW. Knowledge gaps impacting the development of bovine viral diarrhea virus control programs in the United States. J Am Vet Med Assoc 2009;235:1171–9.
48. Grooms DL, Brock KV, Bolin SR, et al. Effect of constant exposure to cattle persistently infected with bovine viral diarrhea virus on morbidity and mortality rates and performance of feedlot cattle. J Am Vet Med Assoc 2014;244:212–24.

49. Fulton RW, Ridpath JF, Ore S, et al. Bovine viral diarrhea virus (BVDV) subgenotypes in diagnostic laboratory accessions: distribution of BVDV1a, 1b, and 2a subgenotypes. Vet Microbiol 2005;111:35–40.

50. Ridpath JF, Fulton RW, Kirkland PD, et al. Prevalence and antigenic differences observed between bovine viral diarrhea virus subgenotypes isolated from cattle in Australia and feedlots in the southwestern United States. J Vet Diagn Invest 2010;22:184–91.

51. Walz PH, Bell TG, Grooms DL, et al. Platelet aggregation responses and virus isolation from platelets in calves experimentally infected with type I or type II bovine viral diarrhea virus. Can J Vet Res 2001;64:241–7.

52. Walz PH, Bell TG, Wells JL, et al. Relationship between degree of viremia and disease manifestations in calves with experimentally induced bovine viral diarrhea virus infection. Am J Vet Res 2001;62:109501103.

53. Janzen ED, Clark EG. The diagnosis of BVD outbreaks in Western Canada. In: Proceedings of the international symposium on bovine viral diarrhea virus. Cornell; 1996. p. 143–58.

54. Carman S, van Dreumel T, Ridpath J, et al. Severe acute bovine viral diarrhea in Ontario, 1993–1995. J Vet Diagn Invest 1998;10:27–35.

55. Hessman BE, Sjeklocha DB, Fulton RF, et al. Acute bovine viral diarrhea associated with extensive mucosal lesions, high morbidity, and mortality in a commercial feedlot. J Vet Diagn Invest 2012;24:397–404.

56. Marshall DJ, Moxley RA, Kelling CL. Distribution of virus and viral antigen in specific pathogen-free calves following inoculation with noncytopathic bovine viral diarrhea virus. Vet Pathol 1996;33:311–8.

57. Ellis JA, West KH, Cortese VS, et al. Lesions and distribution of viral antigen following an experimental infection of young seronegative calves with virulent bovine virus diarrhea virus-type II. Can J Vet Res 1998;62:161–9.

58. Stoffregen B, Bolin SR, Ridpath JF, et al. Morphologic lesions in Type 2 BVDV infections experimentally induced by strain BVDV2-1373 recovered from a field case. Vet Microbiol 2000;77:157–62.

59. Terrell SP, Thomson DU, Wileman BW, et al. A survey to describe current feeder cattle health and well-being program recommendations made by feedlot veterinary consultants in the United States and Canada. Bov Pract 2011;45(2):140–8.

60. Fulton RW, Briggs RE, Ridpath JF, et al. Transmission of bovine viral diarrhea virus 1b to susceptible and vaccinated calves by exposure to persistently infected calves. Can J Vet Res 2005;69:161–9.

61. Theurer M, Larson RL, White BJ. Systematic review and meta-analysis of the effectiveness of commercially available vaccines against bovine herpesvirus, bovine viral diarrhea virus, bovine respiratory syncytial virus, and parainfluenza type 3 virus for mitigation of bovine respiratory disease complex in cattle. J Am Vet Med Assoc 2015;246:126–42.

62. Stilwell G, Matos M, Carolino N, et al. Effect of a quadrivalent vaccine against respiratory virus on the incidence of respiratory disease in weaned beef calves. Prev Vet Med 2008;85:151–7.

63. Makoschey B, Bielsa JM, Oliviero L, et al. Field efficacy of combination vaccines against bovine respiratory pathogens in calves. Acta Vet Hung 2008;56:485–93.

64. Perino LJ, Hunsaker BD. A review of bovine respiratory disease vaccine field efficacy. Bov Pract 1997;31(1):59–66.

65. Nickell JS, White BJ, Larson RL, et al. A simulation model to quantify the value of implementing whole-herd bovine viral diarrhea virus testing strategies in beef cow-calf herds. J Vet Diagn Invest 2011;23:194–205.

66. Academy of Veterinary Consultant position statement on disposal of BVDv PI cattle Available at: http://www.avc-beef.org/Policy/positionstatements.asp. Accessed January 28, 2015.
67. American Association of Bovine Practitioners position statement on disposal of BVDv PI cattle. Available at: http://aabp.org/Members/Documents/PPM-SecE-3.24.2011.pdf#search=%22%20position%20statements%20%22. Accessed January 28, 2015.
68. National Cattlemen's Beef Association. Policy book CH8.5. 2014. p. 46–7. Available at: http://www.beefusa.org/CMDocs/BeefUSA/Issues/2014%20NCBA%20Policy%20Book.pdf. Accessed January 28, 2015.

Feedlot Acute Interstitial Pneumonia

Amelia R. Woolums, DVM, MVSc, PhD

KEYWORDS

- Bovine • Respiratory • Lung injury • 3-Methylindole • Bacteria

KEY POINTS

- Feedlot acute interstitial pneumonia (AIP) is a sporadically occurring respiratory condition of feedlot cattle that is often fatal; death can occur before any signs of disease are recognized.
- Feedlot AIP disproportionately affects heifers and cattle on feed for more than 45 days; more cases occur during hot, dusty weather, but cases can occur at any time.
- Definitive diagnosis of AIP requires histopathologic evaluation of lung tissue; thus, diagnosis based on clinical signs or gross findings alone may be inaccurate.
- No effective treatment of feedlot AIP has been confirmed. Rational therapies include antibiotics effective against common bacterial respiratory pathogens and aspirin or other nonsteroidal anti-inflammatory drugs, administered at label doses.

INTRODUCTION: NATURE OF THE PROBLEM

In feedlot cattle, AIP is a sporadically occurring respiratory condition that is often fatal. Over the years, the disease has been known by other names, including atypical interstitial pneumonia, pulmonary adenomatosis, or dust pneumonia. Although AIP occurs less commonly than shipping fever (fibrinous bronchopneumonia, also known as bovine respiratory disease [BRD]) in North American feedlots, it can have a serious negative impact for individual feedlots, because cattle that have been on feed for greater than 45 days are most often affected, because no treatment is confirmed to be reliably effective, and because multiple cases sometimes occur within a short period of time.

Clinical Definition

Cattle with AIP have a sudden onset of labored breathing. They are often found standing with the head lowered and neck extended, breathing with an open and frothing mouth and with expiratory grunting. Affected cattle may have a basewide stance in

The author has nothing to disclose.
Department of Pathobiology and Population Medicine, College of Veterinary Medicine, Mississippi State University, 240 Wise Center Drive, PO Box 6100, Mississippi State, MS 39762, USA
E-mail address: amelia.woolums@msstate.edu

Vet Clin Food Anim 31 (2015) 381–389
http://dx.doi.org/10.1016/j.cvfa.2015.05.010
0749-0720/15/$ – see front matter © 2015 Elsevier Inc. All rights reserved.

the front limbs (**Fig. 1**). Clinical signs sometimes include fever, but nasal discharge and coughing are not common. If an animal suspected of having AIP is moved for examination or treatment, it is important to move the animal cautiously, because sudden exertion or excitement can precipitate death. Cattle with AIP may be found dead without previous signs of disease having been noticed.

To be precise, AIP is a pathologic definition that can only be confirmed by microscopic (histopathologic) evaluation of lung tissue from an affected individual. A live animal can only be identified to have signs consistent with AIP, because without a lung biopsy AIP cannot be definitively diagnosed in the live animal. In humans and other species with AIP, characteristic clinical signs and diagnostic test results are used to confirm a clinical definition of acute respiratory distress syndrome (ARDS).[1] In other words, AIP is a pathologic diagnosis and ARDS is a clinical diagnosis. Because the term AIP has long been used to reference both antemortem and postmortem cases in feedlot cattle, however, this terminology is used to describe the clinical and pathologic syndrome throughout this article.

Although cattle with AIP exhibit typical clinical signs, these signs are not pathognomonic for AIP. Differential diagnoses for respiratory distress in feedlot cattle include

- Heat stress
- Severe or chronic bronchopneumonia (BRD)
- Anaphylaxis
- Heart failure
- Tracheal edema syndrome
- Necrotic laryngitis

Careful observation may help prioritize the differential diagnoses for a given case. For example, cattle with tracheal edema syndrome or necrotic laryngitis should have prominent noise (stridor) on inspiration. Cattle with heart failure may have peripheral (brisket) edema. During hot weather many feedlot cattle may breathe with an open mouth as part of the normal thermoregulatory process, so open-mouthed breathing alone is not necessarily a sign of respiratory distress.

Because AIP cannot be definitively diagnosed in the live feedlot animal, a diagnosis can only be confirmed by microscopic (histopathologic) evaluation of lung tissue collected at postmortem. Experienced feedlot staff may be able to accurately identify many AIP cases, but even knowledgeable individuals may misdiagnose some AIP cases based on clinical signs or gross pathology alone. Reports indicated that 67%

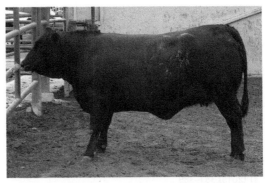

Fig. 1. Feedlot heifer with clinical signs consistent with AIP, including extended neck, frothing at the mouth, and basewide stance in front legs.

to 82% of cattle suspected by experienced individuals to have AIP based on their clinical signs were confirmed by histopathologic evaluation, with the remaining cases confirmed to have BRD or other conditions.[2,3]

Pathology of Acute Interstitial Pneumonia

Grossly, lungs of cattle with AIP remain expanded when the chest is opened, as if they are inflated. Abnormalities are most prominent in the dorsocaudal lung, although the entire lung can be affected.[4] The lung tissue has a firm, rubbery consistency. Individual lung lobules may vary in color from pale pink or gray to brown, dark red, or purple, giving the lung a patchwork quilt or checkerboard appearance (**Fig. 2**).[2,4] Emphysematous bullae or interstitial emphysema may be grossly evident.[2,4] It is important, however, to remember that the presence of grossly evident emphysema does not by itself confirm a diagnosis of AIP. Emphysema can develop after agonal breathing in cattle that die due to a variety of causes.

If a knife is used to cut the lung in cross-section, the cut surface of lung may appear shiny, due to edema; hemorrhage may also be evident. Manual manipulation of the lung often reveals the lobules to be independently movable, because they are separated by edema or emphysema.[3] In some cases, lungs with gross lesions of AIP also have grossly apparent lesions of fibrinous bronchopneumonia (BRD) in the cranial and/or ventral lung, with firm, dark red, gray, or brown lung that has fibrin on the pleural surface.[2,5] In such cases, primary, possibly chronic, bronchopneumonia may have predisposed the animal to development of superimposed (secondary) AIP. This lesion is sometimes referred to as the upstairs-downstairs lesion.

Microscopically, the lesions of AIP include pink homogenous material consisting of proteinaceous fluid (sometimes condensed into hyaline membranes) in the alveoli.[2-4] Neutrophils, macrophages, and sometimes eosinophils infiltrate into alveoli and airways. Edema and hemorrhage may be present in some lobules. These may be the only lesions in cattle that die soon after disease onset (the exudative phase of AIP). In cases of cattle that live longer, proliferation of alveolar type II pneumocytes occurs and is seen microscopically (the proliferative phase of AIP).[2-4] With more time,

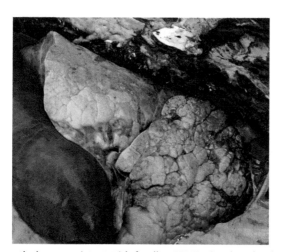

Fig. 2. Gross lung pathology consistent with feedlot AIP. Notice that the dorsocaudal lung is expanded, and individual lobules are clearly demarcated, especially in the cranioventral lung. (*From* Panciera RJ, Confer AW. Pathogenesis and pathology of bovine pneumonia. Vet Clin North Am Food Anim Pract 2010;26:202; with permission.)

inflammatory cells and fibrous tissue may infiltrate the interstitial space. These are the microscopic lesions used to identify AIP.

Although AIP is an acute disease, some cattle also have histopathologic evidence of chronic or past airway injury, including bronchiolitis obliterans.[2,4,6] In 1 study, AIP cases were significantly more likely to have bronchiolitis obliterans than control pen-mates without any history of treatment of lung disease.[2] Bronchiolitis obliterans results from injury to the airway epithelium and could be due to recent or past viral or bacterial infection or injury from pneumotoxins or inhaled irritants. In humans, the lesion can also result from immune-mediated conditions.[7] The frequent occurrence of bronchiolitis obliterans in cases of feedlot AIP may be a clue to the etiology, but the exact cause of the lesion is not known. In some cases, cattle with the definitive histopathologic lesions of AIP also have microscopic lesions consistent with recent or concurrent viral or bacterial lung infection, such as peribronchiolar lymphocytic infiltrate or infiltration of neutrophils into airways or alveoli.

Epidemiology and Risk Factors

In the 2011 US Department of Agriculture *National Animal Health Monitoring System* survey,[8] 72% of all feedlots reported having cattle with AIP, with AIP affecting 2.8% of cattle placed. For comparison, 97% of feedlots reported having cattle with shipping fever (BRD), with BRD affecting 16.2% of cattle placed. A survey of causes of death in yearling feedlot cattle over a single year in 4 western US feedlots revealed AIP in 5.3% of the cattle subjected to necropsy.[4] Mortality risk for AIP ranging from 0.03% to 0.15% of all cattle placed have been reported.[4,9] The majority of AIP cases occur during hot, dusty weather,[3,10] but cases can occur at any time of the year and in any weather.

Compared with fatal shipping fever, cattle die of AIP relatively late in the feeding period[11]; the average number of days on feed at the time of death for cattle with AIP has been reported to range from 114 to 136 days.[2,3,11] Heifers are often disproportionately affected, and in 1 report the odds of an animal with AIP being a heifer were 3.1 times greater than male cattle.[12] In a survey of feedlots to determine risk factors for AIP, however, feedlots where 50% to 75% of placements were heifers did not always report having cases of AIP.[10] Thus, in feedlots where AIP occurs, heifers may be disproportionately affected, but feedlots placing large numbers of heifers do not always see AIP.

Digestive problems may predispose feedlot cattle to AIP. An analysis of health records for 128,500 feedlot cattle collected over 18 months showed that the incidence of AIP was approximately 70% greater in pens where at least 1 digestive death occurred compared with pens where a digestive death did not occur.[13] AIP does not, however, seem to result from acidosis; cattle with feedlot AIP have been found to have higher ruminal pH values than expected for cattle adapted to a high concentrated diet. Ruminal pH in AIP cases ranged from 5.6 to 7.2 in 1 study[2] and from 4.9 to 7.4 in another,[14] whereas the ruminal pH of cattle adapted to a high concentrate diet is typically approximately 5.5 to 5.6.[15] Many proteins are relatively basic; therefore, the high ruminal pH could be related to abnormal protein metabolism. The relatively high ruminal pH, however, could also be caused by anorexia. The concept that abnormal ruminal protein metabolism may contribute to feedlot AIP is also supported by a small study that found increased ammonia levels in the ruminal gas cap of cattle with AIP.[16]

A survey of US feedlots undertaken to characterize risk factors for feedlot AIP[10] found that feedlots in northern states (Nebraska, Utah, Idaho, South Dakota, North Dakota, Montana, and Washington) were less likely to recognize AIP as a cause of morbidity and mortality than feedlots in other states, with 66% of northern feedlots recognizing AIP versus 94% of feedlots in other regions (P<.01). Larger feedlots were more likely to recognize AIP; 90% of responding feedlots that placed 10,000 or more cattle annually reported AIP as a cause of morbidity and mortality compared with 62% of feedlots placing fewer than 10,000 head annually (P<.01). Feedlots that vaccinated more than 95% of their cattle against *Mannheimia haemolytica* with or without *Pasteurella multocida* were less likely to report seeing AIP cases compared with feedlots vaccinating 95% or fewer of their cattle (P<.001). The significance of the relationship between *Mannheimia/Pasteurella* vaccination and AIP is not known. Because a trend toward increased recognition of AIP by feedlots placing more yearling cattle was also identified in the survey, the relationship between *Mannheimia/Pasteurella* vaccination and decreased recognition of AIP may have been because AIP was less common in feedlots placing younger cattle, where vaccination against *Mannheimia/Pasteurella* was likely more common.

Etiology

AIP occurs after injury to alveolar epithelial cells; therefore, cattle with feedlot AIP have been exposed to something that injures these cells. The exact cause of this injury is usually not known. In cattle outside of feedlots, pneumotoxic compounds, such as 3-methylindole (3-MI), produced by ruminal metabolism of L-tryptophan in green forage[17] are known to cause injury to bronchiolar and alveolar epithelial cells, leading to AIP. Metabolites of 3-MI, such as 3-methyleneindolenine, bind to cellular proteins and nucleic acids, leading to cellular dysfunction and death. Pneumotoxins in moldy sweet potatoes[18] and perilla mint[19] likewise cause AIP by direct cellular injury. Other feeds, including turnip tops, moldy hay, and individual batches of silage, have been associated with AIP outbreaks, but the causative components of these feeds is not known. Toxic gases, such as nitrogen dioxide, zinc oxide, or chlorine gas, can cause AIP, but in most cases feedlot cattle are unlikely to be exposed to concentrations of these gases sufficient to cause disease. Smoke inhalation can also cause AIP, and exposure is usually obvious.

Although the exact cause of feedlot AIP is not known, research undertaken to determine the cause has identified the following factors to be associated with the disease in one or more reports:

- 3-MI and metabolites of 3-MI[3,12]
  - ○ Possible sources: tryptophan in ration components, disrupted ruminal protein metabolism
- Melengestrol acetate (MGA)[20,21]
- Bovine respiratory syncytial virus (BRSV) infection[2,22]
- Bacterial pneumonia[2,9]
- Airway epithelial cell injury (bronchiolitis obliterans)[2,4,6]
  - ○ Possible causes: recent or past bacterial or viral infection, inhalation of dust or other irritants, lung inflammatory processes
- Hot weather[2–4]
- Dusty conditions[3,4]

It is likely that in many cases, 2 or more of these factors interact to induce AIP. For example, experimental exposure of cattle to BRSV with 3-MI has been shown to cause lung lesions of significantly increased severity compared with those seen in cattle exposed to BRSV or 3-MI alone.[23] Taken together, the available information suggests that (1) factors related to the formulation or delivery of the diet or rumen metabolism of dietary components and/or (2) viral or bacterial respiratory infection are likely the most important factors contributing to the development of most cases of feedlot AIP.

Numerous reports suggest that more AIP cases occur during hot or dusty weather, but it is not clear how weather influences AIP incidence risk. Perhaps hot or dusty weather simply puts the respiratory system under more pressure when it is already primed for AIP by 1 or more of the factors listed previously, pushing more cattle to a tipping point that leads to disease. Exposure of sheep or goats to repeated doses of aerosolized feedlot dust containing microorganisms and endotoxin did not lead to AIP,[24,25] and exposure to M haemolytica or P multocida did not induce serious lung disease in goats exposed to aerosolized feedlot dust.[25] Moreover, tracheal instillation of spores of fungi commonly found in feedlot dust did not induce AIP in goats.[26] These studies suggest that feedlot dust exposure alone is unlikely to cause AIP.

THERAPEUTIC OPTIONS

Evidence-based guidelines for treatment of feedlot AIP are lacking. There are currently no specific treatments for humans with the clinical syndrome ARDS, likely due to AIP[27,28]; current recommendations for treatment of humans with ARDS include rigorous supportive care, with certain mechanical ventilation strategies most commonly cited as improving outcomes. Feedlot cattle with AIP are not candidates for mechanical ventilation.

In humans, β-adrenergic agonists, high-dose or moderate-dose corticosteroids, neutrophil elastase inhibitors, and a variety of other therapies have been tested but have failed to improve outcomes in patients with ARDS.[28] Low doses of corticosteroids seem beneficial, but repeated daily treatments for 1 to 4 weeks are used[29]; such a regimen is not likely feasible for use in feedlot cattle.

Although no specific therapies are proved effective in cattle with feedlot AIP, and no drugs are labeled for the treatment of feedlot AIP, it is rational to treat cattle suspected of having AIP with drugs that address the lesions known to occur in affected lungs, namely, cellular injury, inflammation, and, in some cases, bacterial infection. Additionally, because antemortem case definition is not perfectly accurate, it is rational to treat apparent AIP cases, because some may actually have bacterial bronchopneumonia or other respiratory disease, instead of AIP. Thus treatments most commonly recommended include

- Label dose of antibiotics appropriate for treatment of M haemolytica and P multocida
  - Consider using products with short withdrawal times in cattle late in the feeding period that may survive until harvest
- Label dose of nonsteroidal anti-inflammatory drugs, in particular aspirin

Because cattle with AIP may die suddenly, and because treatment may not be effective, emergency slaughter of AIP cases when they are first identified may be the best course of action.[3,13]

Prevention of Feedlot Acute Interstitial Pneumonia

Strong scientific support for any recommendation to prevent feedlot AIP is lacking. Monensin decreases the metabolism of tryptophan to 3-MI by Lactobacillus sp in the rumen; thus, feeding monensin can help prevent AIP associated with a sudden transition to lush forage, and feeding monensin may also help control feedlot AIP. Feedlot cattle fed rations, however, including monensin sometimes develop AIP.[2,30]

Because free radical scavengers can reduce the toxicity of metabolites of 3-MI, both vitamin E[30,31] and the glutathione precursor cysteine (provided as feather meal)[30] have been administered to decrease rates of AIP or to improve growth and health in cattle at risk for AIP. No clear beneficial effect of these treatments, however, has been identified.

Likewise, although aspirin is theoretically beneficial because it can inhibit function of prostaglandin H synthetase, which can generate toxic metabolites from 3-MI,[32] a clear protective effect against AIP has not been demonstrated.[31,33] It has been claimed, however, that aspirin treatment of cattle with clinical signs of AIP is associated with longer survival.[34]

Removal of MGA from the diets of heifers has been reported to decrease rates of AIP.[35] In a subsequent clinical trial, these researchers found no difference in death loss in pens of heifers fed MGA compared with pens of heifers not fed MGA; however, rates of emergency slaughter (due to clinical signs consistent with AIP) for heifers fed MGA were more than 3 times higher than those for heifers not fed MGA.[21] Other investigators have suggested, however, that erratic consumption of MGA, leading to estrus, with related hormonal changes, decreased feed intake, and resulting digestive changes, may actually cause AIP.[13] This line of reasoning suggests that inadequate MGA consumption leads to AIP. If MGA does contribute to the pathogenesis of AIP, its role is not clear; it has been speculated to increase production of 3-MI through multiple possible pathways.

Given the list of factors associated with feedlot AIP, it is rational to consider the following interventions to decrease occurrence of the disease:

- Ensure that rations are formulated, mixed, and delivered consistently.
- Ensure that monensin is included at the highest appropriate dose.
- Review MGA use if AIP in heifers is a problem.
  - Ensure consistent intake, or consider removing from ration (expert views are mixed on the role of MGA).
- Institute practices to decrease dust and minimize heat stress.
  - Particular focus on pens of long-fed animals may be most efficient.
- Ensure timely identification and treatment of cattle with signs of BRD, which may predispose cattle to later develop AIP.

CLINICAL OUTCOMES

Case fatality and chronic rates for cattle identified with signs of AIP have not been published, but the reported use of emergency slaughter to handle cases suggests that feedlots do not find therapy to be rewarding. Because it is not possible to make a definitive antemortem diagnosis of AIP in the feedlot setting, it is difficult to know whether cattle that survive an apparent episode of AIP truly had AIP. Humans that survive episodes of ARDS can have long-term debilitation that has a negative impact on quality of life.[27]

SUMMARY

Feedlot AIP is a sporadically occurring respiratory condition of feedlot cattle that is often fatal, and death can occur before any signs of disease are recognized. Feedlot AIP most often affects cattle on feed for more than 45 days, and heifers are often disproportionately affected. More cases occur during hot, dusty weather, but cases can occur at any time. The exact cause in feedlot cattle is usually not known. Taken together, the available information suggests that (1) factors related to the formulation or delivery of the diet or rumen metabolism of dietary components and/or (2) viral or bacterial respiratory infection is likely the most important factor contributing to the development of most cases of feedlot AIP. No effective treatment of feedlot AIP has been confirmed. Rational therapies include antibiotics effective against common bacterial respiratory pathogens and aspirin or other nonsteroidal anti-inflammatory drugs, administered at label doses. Effective preventive strategies are not well defined; recommended practices include efforts to control dust and prevent heat stress in long-fed cattle; to ensure consistent formulation, mixing, and delivery of feed; and to identify and treat infectious BRD in a timely manner, because BRD may predispose cattle to later develop AIP.[27]

REFERENCES

1. Mukhopadhyay S, Parambil JG. Acute interstitial pneumonia (AIP): relationship to Hamman-Rich syndrome, diffuse alveolar damage (DAD), and acute respiratory distress syndrome (ARDS). Semin Respir Crit Care Med 2012;33(5):476–85.
2. Woolums AR, Mason GL, Hawkins LL, et al. Microbiologic findings in feedlot cattle with acute interstitial pneumonia. Am J Vet Res 2004;65(11):1525–32.
3. Ayroud M, Popp JD, VanderKop MA, et al. Characterization of acute interstitial pneumonia in cattle in southern Alberta feedyards. Can Vet J 2000;41(7):547–54.
4. Jensen R, Pierson RE, Braddy PM, et al. Atypical interstitial pneumonia in yearling feedlot cattle. J Am Vet Med Assoc 1976;169(5):507–10.
5. Panciera RJ, Confer AW. Pathogenesis and pathology of bovine pneumonia. Vet Clin North Am Food Anim Pract 2010;26(2):191–214.
6. Sorden SD, Kerr RW, Janzen ED. Interstitial pneumonia in feedlot cattle: concurrent lesions and lack of immunohistochemical evidence for bovine respiratory syncytial virus infection. J Vet Diagn Invest 2000;12(6):510–7.
7. Barker AF, Bergeron A, Rom WN, et al. Obliterative bronchiolitis. N Engl J Med 2014;370(19):1820–8.
8. USDA. Feedlot 2011 Part IV: health and health management on U.S. feedlots with a capacity of 1,000 or more head. Ft Collins (CO): USDA-APHIS-VS-CEAH-NAHMS; 2011.
9. Hjerpe CA. Clinical management of respiratory disease in feedlot cattle. Vet Clin North Am Large Anim Pract 1983;5(1):119–42.
10. Woolums AR, Loneragan GH, Hawkins LL, et al. A survey of the relationship between management practices and risk of acute interstitial pneumonia at U.S. feedlots. Bov Pract 2005;39:125.
11. Loneragan GH, Gould DH, Mason GL, et al. Involvement of microbial respiratory pathogens in acute interstitial pneumonia in feedlot cattle. Am J Vet Res 2001; 62(10):1519–24.
12. Loneragan GH, Gould DH, Mason GL, et al. Association of 3-methyleneindolenine, a toxic metabolite of 3-methylindole, with acute interstitial pneumonia in feedlot cattle. Am J Vet Res 2001;62(10):1525–30.
13. Loneragan GH. Epidemiological characteristics of AIP in feedlot cattle. Proc Acad Vet Consult. Summer Meeting:1. Colorado Springs, August 1–3, 2002.
14. Miles DG, Hoffman BW, Rogers KC, et al. Diagnosis of digestive deaths. J Anim Sci 1998;76(1):320–2.
15. Fulton WR, Klopfenstein TJ, Britton RA. Adaptation to high concentrate diets by beef cattle. I. Adaptation to corn and wheat diets. J Anim Sci 1979;49:775.
16. Loneragan GH, Gould DH. Atypical interstitial pneumonia in U.S. feedlots. Proc Acad Vet Consult. Winter Meeting:1. Denver, December 2–4, 1999.
17. Dickinson EO, Spencer GR, Gorham JR. Experimental induction of an acute respiratory syndrome in cattle resembling bovine pulmonary emphysema. Vet Rec 1967;80(16):487–9.

18. Peckham JC, Mitchell FE, Jones OH Jr, et al. Atypical interstitial pneumonia in cattle fed moldy sweet potatoes. J Am Vet Med Assoc 1972;160(2):169–72.
19. Kerr LA, Johnson BJ, Burrows GE. Intoxication of cattle by Perilla frutescens (purple mint). Vet Hum Toxicol 1986;28(5):412–6.
20. Popp JD, McAllister TA, Kastelic JP, et al. Effect of melengestrol acetate on development of 3-methylindole-induced pulmonary edema and emphysema in sheep. Can J Vet Res 1998;62(4):268–74.
21. Stanford K, McAllister TA, Ayroud M, et al. Effect of dietary melengestrol acetate on the incidence of acute interstitial pneumonia in feedlot heifers. Can J Vet Res 2006;70(3):218–25.
22. Collins JK, Jensen R, Smith GH, et al. Association of bovine respiratory syncytial virus with atypical interstitial pneumonia in feedlot cattle. Am J Vet Res 1988;49(7):1045–9.
23. Bingham HR, Morley PS, Wittum TE, et al. Synergistic effects of concurrent challenge with bovine respiratory syncytial virus and 3-methylindole in calves. Am J Vet Res 1999;60(5):563–70.
24. Purdy CW, Straus DC, Chirase N, et al. Effects of aerosolized feedyard dust that contains natural endotoxins on adult sheep. Am J Vet Res 2002;63(1):28–35.
25. Purdy CW, Straus DC, Chirase N, et al. Effects of aerosolized dust in goats on lung clearance of Pasteurella and Mannheimia species. Curr Microbiol 2003; 46(3):174–9.
26. Purdy CW, Layton RC, Straus DC, et al. Virulence of fungal spores determined by tracheal inoculation of goats following inhalation of aerosolized sterile feedyard dust. Am J Vet Res 2005;66(4):615–22.
27. Carlucci M, Graf N, Simmons JQ, et al. Effective management of ARDS. Nurse Pract 2014;39(12):35–40.
28. Boyle AJ, Mac Sweeney R, McAuley DF. Pharmacological treatments in ARDS; a state-of-the-art update. BMC Med 2013;11:166.
29. Tang BM, Craig JC, Eslick GD, et al. Use of corticosteroids in acute lung injury and acute respiratory distress syndrome: a systematic review and meta-analysis. Crit Care Med 2009;37(5):1594–603.
30. Stanford K, McAllister TA, Ayroud M, et al. Acute interstitial pneumonia in feedlot cattle: effects of feeding feather meal or vitamin E. Can J Vet Res 2007;71(2): 152–6.
31. Loneragan GH, Morley PS, Wagner JJ, et al. Effects of feeding aspirin and supplemental vitamin E on plasma concentrations of 3-methylindole, 3-methylenein-dolenine-adduct concentrations in blood and pulmonary tissues, lung lesions, and growth performance in feedlot cattle. Am J Vet Res 2002;63(12):1641–7.
32. Bray TM, Emmerson KS. Putative Mechanisms of Toxicity of 3-Methylindole - from Free-Radical to Pneumotoxicosis. Annu Rev Pharmacol 1994;34:91–115.
33. Bingham HR, Wittum TE, Morley PS, et al. Evaluation of the ability of orally administered aspirin to mitigate effects of 3-methylindole in feedlot cattle. Am J Vet Res 2000;61(10):1209–13.
34. McAllister T. Characterization of atypical interstitial pneumonia in feedlot cattle in southern Alberta. Proc Acad Vet Consult. Spring Meeting. Oklahoma City (OK), April 5–7, 2007. p. 13–22.
35. Woolums AR, McAllister TA, Loneragan GH, et al. Etiology of acute interstitial pneumonia in feedlot cattle: noninfectious causes. Compend Cont Educ Pract Vet 2001;23:S86–93.

Investigating Outbreaks of Disease or Impaired Productivity in Feedlot Cattle

David R. Smith, DVM, PhD

KEYWORDS

- Feedlot • Cattle • Disease • Outbreak investigation • Impaired productivity

KEY POINTS

- Outbreaks are an unexpected increase in morbidity, mortality, or impaired productivity.
- The reasons for investigating outbreaks of disease or impaired productivity are to reduce losses from existing cases, prevent additional cases, and understand how future outbreaks can be avoided.
- Outbreak investigations are more likely to be successful if an orderly process of investigation is followed using logic based on causal theory.
- Outbreaks are often the result of decisions and actions taken within the system, even though those actions may have taken place long ago or in a different location from the current problem.
- The investigation should be followed up with a clearly written report, which includes recommendations for measurable actions.

INTRODUCTION

The goal of a feedlot production system is to receive cattle to feed and finish, then market the cattle for harvest and processing into beef. Most cattle move through this system without health problems or impairment of productivity. Some feedlot cattle do become ill or unproductive. Disease and poor growth performance are expected to occur at some level of frequency in most feedlots.[1] The direct cause of disease in feedlot cattle may be well known and well characterized, although sometimes it is not. Even with excellent understanding of the pathophysiology of the disease, it may still be a challenge to understand what factors in the production system have

The author has no conflicts of interest to disclose.
A contribution of the Beef Cattle Population Health and Reproduction Program at Mississippi State University. Supported by the Mikell and Mary Cheek Hall Davis Endowment for Beef Cattle Health and Reproduction.
Department of Pathobiology and Population Medicine, College of Veterinary Medicine, Mississippi State University, PO Box 6100, 240 Wise Center Drive, Mississippi State, MS 39762, USA
E-mail address: david.smith@msstate.edu

led to the current problem.[2] Understanding what has gone wrong and how to remedy the situation may be particularly important when the disease occurs at an unexpectedly high rate.

An outbreak is defined as an unexpected increase in morbidity, mortality, or impaired productivity.[3–5] Outbreaks of disease or impaired productivity are indications that something in the production system is out of control.[6] Often, the root cause of an outbreak relates to a change in human actions or decisions, sometimes far removed in time or space from the clinical occurrence of the problem.[7]

IMPORTANT CONCEPTS
Causal Reasoning

Outbreak investigations are studies of causation. In conducting the investigation, we are trying to understand what caused the disease or impaired productivity to occur and hoping to prevent future problems. It is not easy to conduct an investigation that solves the problem, even if we do come to understand the disease process, because causal inference is complicated.

By the nature of their training in infectious diseases, with emphasis placed on individual animal medicine, veterinarians often spend considerable time and money trying to identify a pathogen to blame for health problems. Sometimes, knowing the pathogen(s) involved in a disease outbreak can useful. For example, it is useful to know that recent feedlot deaths were associated with infection with *Clostridium chauvoei* or *Listeria monocytogenes*. However, that causal information alone does not explain why cattle deaths suddenly occur from either of these widely distributed environmental source pathogens. Outbreak investigations can become sidetracked, and both human and capital resources consumed, in the sole pursuit of a causative agent, rather than identifying more useful explanations for the outbreak. Knowing the name of the causative agent may provide an explanation for the observed disease and might provide therapeutic insight. However, that knowledge rarely explains the course of events that led to the outbreak or provides a solution for preventing future problems.

Each factor that contributes to the development of disease is a component cause. Disease is observed when component causes add up to complete a sufficient cause.[8] Without a sufficient cause being completed, there is no observation of disease. That factor explains why we might recover *Mannheimia hemolytica* from a deep nasopharyngeal swab of a calf without respiratory disease, or why 1 feedlot manager might observe greater rates of respiratory disease with changes in the weather and another after a feed change. Each outbreak of respiratory disease is the result of the completion of a sufficient cause, which might have also included the presence of viral and bacterial pathogens, a certain state of immunity, or other component causes of respiratory disease in cattle that we fail to understand. In general, the objective of an outbreak investigation is to determine which potential component causes (eg, causal factors or risk factors) contribute to the completion of a sufficient cause. Removing 1 or more component causes prevents the expression of disease. Manageable component causes are called key determinants. In this example, it is rarely possible to control the weather, so managing feed changes may be the key determinant. Sometimes, key determinants are far removed in time or place from the immediate problem.

We may be more successful meeting the objectives of a field investigation if we can identify how certain actions or decisions inherent to the production system led up to (caused) the problem. For example, solutions are more likely to come from knowing that the blackleg cases occurred in pens in which the pen surface had recently been dug up or scraped aggressively, or that *Listeria* cases coincided with opening a new silage bunker. Knowing that personnel changes or changes in arrival processing practices preceded the problem may be more useful than naming an agent. The science of system dynamics holds promise in helping veterinarians understand how actions and decisions far removed from the immediate problem could be a cause of the problem.[7] For example, a large regional drought could cause cow-calf producers to decide to wean calves early, seek feedlot pens to house cows, or to depopulate their herds, all of which may have effects on feedlot management and health. Small cow-calf producers may decide not to dehorn, castrate, vaccinate, or deworm calves on the farm because they lack facilities or fail to recognize an economic signal to do so. Decisions made months ago at a farm, possibly hundreds of miles away, may result in increased morbidity and mortality in the feedlot.[9]

Even although the goal of outbreak investigation is to understand what caused the outbreak and determine what to do about it, it is not easy, and perhaps impossible, to prove that 1 thing causes another. Philosophers continue to debate the subject,[10] as do epidemiologists.[8,11–15] However, Koch,[16] Hill,[17] Susser,[18] and Evans[19] have each discussed guidelines for thinking about causation in the health sciences. Each makes a case for causal relationships having characteristics such that the proposed cause (1) precedes the outcome, (2) has a strong association with the outcome, (3) has been associated with the outcome in more than 1 study, (4) shows a dose effect with the outcome, and (5) has consistency with current knowledge. Although these criteria may guide our thinking in an outbreak investigation, none is necessary or sufficient for establishing that a causal relationship exists. Beyond these criteria, our own cognitive biases may make it difficult to draw the correct conclusions from our observations during an outbreak investigation.[20] For example, we may fail to recognize a key finding or observation because it did not fit our framework of knowledge about disease causation. Outbreak investigations serve a practical purpose to identify reasonable actions to reduce current losses and prevent future outbreaks. If action to prevent a potential cause seems prudent and comes at little cost, then, there is little harm in taking it, even in the absence of complete causal evidence. However, if the cost of the action is potentially high, then, a higher standard of causal reasoning is justified.

Level of Action

The factors responsible for outbreaks of disease or impaired productivity in feedlot cattle might occur at different levels of organization. For example, the factor may be acting at the level of the individual, pen, or feedlot. Some causal factors act at the individual level. For example, a growth-promoting implant affects the growth potential of individual cattle.[21] Implanting a given steer has negligible effect on other steers in the pen (although when the implanted steer gets up to eat, it may stimulate other cattle to also go to the bunk to eat). On the other hand, some factors have a stronger group effect. For example, the energy density of the ration delivered to the feedbunk is likely to affect the entire group similarly (although individual cattle may have eating patterns that are more likely to lead to acidosis).[22] Group and individual levels of action often occur at the same time. It is likely that a particular viral infection would have a strong group-level effect, such that if 1 animal in a pen has a viral infection, then, most cattle in the pen have the same viral infection. However, there may be characteristics of individual cattle, such as previous immunity, that mean that a sufficient cause is not always completed and therefore clinical signs are observed only in certain cattle. Many measures of health and performance are primarily affected at the feedlot level because of the unique combination of natural resources, human resources, and capital represented by a particular feeding operation. For example, cattle within a feedlot may have similar patterns of health and performance because of management decisions that occur at the feedlot level. Some health problems are regional in occurrence such that the level of action may have regional or geopolitical levels of action.

Herd immunity is an important example of a group-level determinant of disease. Herd immunity occurs when there is a sufficiently large proportion of the group having individual protective immunity against a pathogen to prevent its transmission to individuals that lack protective immunity. In a population in which herd immunity may play a protective role, it may not be sufficient to know an individual's immune status; it may be necessary to interpret an individual's immune status in the context of the immune status of others. Although the concept of herd immunity is important and likely comes into play in cattle populations, the proportion of a group that must have protective immunity to prevent transmission of common feedlot pathogens has not been determined.[23]

WHY INVESTIGATE OUTBREAKS

Typically, a cattle feeder might be motivated to request an outbreak investigation to (1) reduce the losses associated with existing cases and (2) prevent new cases from occurring.[5] However, sometimes, the outbreak will have run its course before an investigation has been initiated. In that circumstance, the justification for investigating the problem is to understand the decisions, actions, and behaviors that led to the outbreak, so that future outbreaks can be prevented. This latter justification of understanding how factors in the system lead to the problem should be a goal of any disease outbreak investigation.

HOW TO INVESTIGATE AN OUTBREAK OF DISEASE OR IMPAIRED PRODUCTIVITY
Steps of an Outbreak Investigation

Outbreak investigations should be conducted in an orderly and logical process.[23]

1. Interview key individuals, including owners, caretakers, veterinarians, nutritionists, and other stakeholders
2. Confirm the clinical diagnosis to ensure that affected individuals receive appropriate care and treatment
3. Make a systems-level diagnosis and identify the factors responsible for the outbreak
4. Develop a strategic plan to prevent new cases or future outbreaks
5. Clearly communicate the results of the investigation and the recommendations to all key individuals
6. Develop a system of record keeping to document that the recommendations were implemented and to evaluate whether the changes were successful in reducing or eliminating the problem

Risk assessment is an approach for (1) evaluating the probability of potential hazards (opportunities) and the costs (benefits) should they occur (termed risk analysis); (2) determining what actions and costs are involved in mitigating those hazards (termed risk management); and (3) communicating the plan to team members and keeping records to document what was done and whether those actions were successful (termed risk communication). In the context of risk assessment, steps 1 to 3 of the outbreak investigation are risk analysis, step 4 is risk management, and steps 5 and 6 are risk communication and documentation.

Early in the course of an outbreak investigation, the key individuals should be identified, interviewed, and contact information gathered. Often, it is the feedlot owner or manager who has asked for assistance, but there may be others with important information unknown to the owner or manager. These key individuals may include feedlot personnel, nutritionists, feed salesmen, and other veterinarians.

The clinical diagnosis of affected cattle should be verified by physical examination and appropriate diagnostic testing. It is also important to reduce ongoing losses by verifying that treatments given to affected cattle are medically appropriate. Determine, through history and records analysis, that this is an outbreak. Sometimes, what is perceived as an outbreak is really a sudden awareness on the owner's or caretaker's part of a disease process that has been ongoing for some time. Be aware that the owner's or manager's complaint might be expressed as their own perception of the problem, but their evaluation may not be representative of the true situation. For example, any number of disease syndromes might be the problem that the manager believes has led to poor performance, although the real cause of reduced gains is an inaccurate scale on the feed truck.

As early as possible, collect diagnostic specimens from the affected cattle and their environment, even if they may not be submitted. Feed components, water, and other environmental sources of microbial or toxic elements may change with the passage of time, making it critical to collect these time-sensitive samples for later analysis if there is any suspicion that these sources may be a cause of the problem.

A critical component of any disease outbreak investigation is specifying what a case is and what it is not.[5] The case definition may mirror the clinical diagnosis, but sometimes, the definition of a case is broader than a single clinical problem. For example, a case definition that might point to the involvement of bovine viral diarrhea virus might include several clinical presentations. Having reasonable specificity in the case definition is important to prevent trying to find a single solution to more than 1 problem. However, if the case definition is overspecified, confusion may result because only part of the problem is being investigated. The process of defining a case may be an iterative one as more is learned about the outbreak.

Classifying a recorded clinical illness appropriately as a case or noncase can be confusing for several reasons. Some cases of the same problem may be coded or recorded differently (eg, diarrhea vs scours). The recorded event might be too specific or not specific enough (eg, recorded as scours, not coccidiosis). Also, it may be important to clarify if a recorded case is (1) an animal pulled by a pen rider for signs of the disease; (2) a diagnosis confirmed by the hospital crew (eg, a pneumonia pull meeting a body temperature requirement); or (3) an animal receiving treatment of the disease. Ideally, all 3 events would be recorded. Definitions for recovery are also important to determine when an animal is at risk to become a case again. The definitions for recovery, relapse, and reinfection should be based on the pathophysiology of the disease. To the author's knowledge, no standard definitions exist for recovery, relapse, or reinfection for the common diseases of cattle.

Equally as important as having an appropriate case definition is defining the population at risk to become a case. For example, if the problem is postcastration complications, then, only cattle that have been castrated are at risk for the disease. If the case definition is postcastration complications in calves that were castrated by feedlot personnel, then, the population at risk is only calves castrated at the feedlot. Similarly, the at-risk population for dystocia in the feedlot may be intact heifers in the feedlot but might more specifically be pregnant heifers in the feedlot.

Describing Outbreaks

Much of the art and science of medicine is about developing skill in pattern recognition. This factor may be especially true in outbreak investigations. Recognizing patterns helps us formulate causal hypotheses. We try to recognize patterns of disease or impaired productivity by describing the outbreak by subject, place, or time; to know who got sick, when, and where.

Subjects may be individual cattle with additional information available, or there may be group-level information (eg, pens of cattle, or the entire feedlot) depending on the level of action. The place is the physical location of affected cattle. It may be useful to plot on a map where cases have occurred, because the distribution of cases by location may provide clues to the disease process. Time can be according to the calendar or according to a relevant starting point. For example, we might be interested in how many cases occurred in July, or how many cases occurred within 30 days of arrival in the feedlot. It may be helpful to graphically portray information about subject and time as a frequency histogram. When counts of cases are plotted by calendar time, the frequency histogram is known as an epidemic curve (**Fig. 1**).

Outbreaks may occur because of a point-source exposure to an infectious or toxic agent. Point-source outbreaks are characterized by a rapid increase in incidence and, often, rapid resolution. Some point-source outbreaks become propagated epidemics if secondary cases continue to occur or if the source of exposure is ongoing. Propagated epidemics are characterized by new cases continuing to occur for a long period.[24] The tactics used to prevent new cases may differ depending on the type of outbreak. For example, the approach may be to remove the source of exposure, or it may be to isolate cases to prevent secondary transmission. Sometimes, the distinction between point-source and propagated outbreaks is not obvious. However, graphing an epidemic curve may still be helpful in understanding the infection dynamics within the population.

Outbreaks should be described using standardized statistics for describing disease events.[25] Prevalence is usually the easiest calculated measure of disease in a population. It is the number of animals with the disease of concern divided by the number of animals in the population, all measured at a single point in time. For example, if you count 30 lame steers in a pen of 150, then, the prevalence of lameness is 20%. Prevalence is a function of incidence and duration of infection. If either incidence or duration increases, so does prevalence. Because prevalence is a function of 2 other statistics, interpreting changes in prevalence can be difficult. For example, if prevalence decreases after changing the treatment regimen, it may be because cattle are recovering or because cattle are dying more rapidly. Similarly, prevalence of disease might paradoxically increase with a successful treatment because the mortality has decreased.

Incidence is the preferred measure to describe the driving force of disease in a population. As a general definition, incidence is the rate of new cases divided by the population at risk for some period. The numerator of incidence is always the number of new cases in a period. Incidence statistics are named according to the method of calculating the denominator. The denominator for cumulative incidence is typically the number of subjects at risk in the population at the beginning of the period of observation (**Fig. 2**). Consider the feedlot pen described earlier with 30 lame steers in a lot of 150. If 20 additional steers become lame in the next 30 days, then, the 30-day cumulative incidence of lameness is 20/120, or 17% per month. This simple calculation of cumulative incidence assumes that the 30 cattle already lame are no longer at risk to become a new case of lameness; that assumption may not be valid. Calculating incidence can be confusing because of the challenge of defining the population at risk. Given that cattle have 4 legs, a lameness in 1 leg does not prevent lameness in another, so, the animal may continue to be at risk for lameness in another leg. The same can be said for digits. Even for a lameness in 1 leg, there is the question of when that injury is healed and the leg is again at risk.

In populations with dynamic changes in population counts, such as feedyards, the population at risk at the beginning of the period may not be the best estimate of the

	A	B	C	D	E	F
1	Count		244	steers		
2	Arrival		9/6/2013			
3	interval		7	days		
4						
5			BRD	All	BRD	BRD
6			Cases	Deaths	at risk	Cum Inc
7	and earlier	9/5	0	0	244	0
8	9/6	9/12	41	4	244	0.17
9	9/13	9/19	56	7	199	0.28
10	9/20	9/26	32	4	136	0.24
11	9/27	10/3	20	4	100	0.20
12	10/4	10/10	13	0	76	0.17
13	10/11	10/17	9	3	63	0.14
14	10/18	10/24	5	1	51	0.10
15	10/25	10/31	0	6	45	0.00

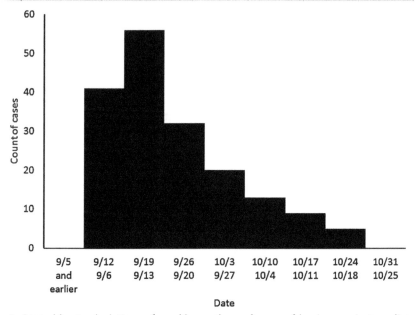

Fig. 1. Spreadsheet calculations of weekly numbers of cases of bovine respiratory disease (BRD), deaths, and population at risk for BRD from 244 steers after receiving, with epidemic curve. Cum Inc, cumulative incidence.

at-risk population. The denominator of incidence density is the sum of time (eg, days) that each animal in the population is at risk. In a feedlot, the days at risk might be the number of days elapsing from the time the animal enters the pen until it is sold, culled, dies, or develops the disease of interest. Calculating incidence density requires that the dates of these events are recorded. The denominator of incidence density has units of subject-time (Fig. 3).

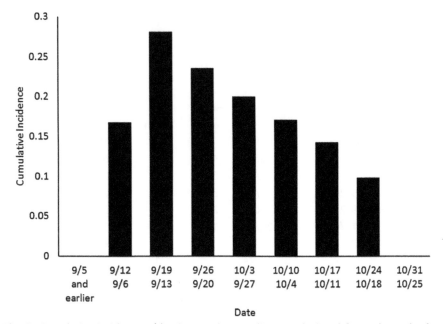

Fig. 2. Cumulative incidence of bovine respiratory disease calculated for each week after receiving from 244 steers corresponding to epidemic curve in **Fig. 1**.

The attack rate is a measurement of incidence particularly useful for outbreaks of short duration. The attack rate is the cumulative incidence for the duration of the outbreak. Often, attack rates are calculated separately for animals with each potential exposure. The exposure with the highest attack rate may be presumed to be an important component cause in the outbreak.

The case fatality rate is useful for describing prognosis or treatment efficacy of cases. Case fatality rate is the number of deaths per case of a particular disease.

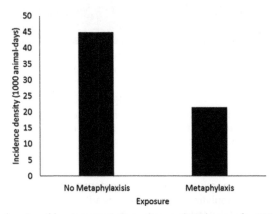

Fig. 3. Incidence density of bovine respiratory disease (BRD) cases for 123 steers treated on arrival with an injectable antibiotic (metaphylaxis) and 121 steers not treated on arrival (no metaphylaxis). The relative risk for BRD for no metaphylactic treatment compared with treatment was 2.1.

The case fatality rate should be expressed for cases occurring over a relevant period. Related, self-explanatory calculations are case recovery rate and case chronicity rate.

The proportional morbidity (or mortality) is a measure of the relative impact of a disease on the total load of sickness (or death) in the population. The proportional morbidity is the number of cases of a particular disease divided by the total number of cases over a unit of time. In an outbreak investigation, this statistic helps put the problem of concern into context with the occurrence of other problems. Changes in proportional morbidity are difficult to interpret. Everything else being equal, as 1 illness decreases, the proportional morbidity of all others must, by definition, increase.

DRAWING CAUSAL CONCLUSIONS

In the process of outbreak investigation, we want to try to describe the relationships between potential risk factors and the outcome of concern to infer causation. This goal is commonly achieved by following causal reasoning and measuring strength of association.

Outbreak investigations in cattle feedlots are frequently qualitative rather than quantitative, because quantitative data (eg, health outcomes relatable to potential risk factors) are not readily available for analysis. This situation is unfortunate, because it often means that feedlot health and performance data were recorded for business purposes, such as billing, but not in a fashion that allows timely or cost-effective analysis of measured health outcomes. Qualitative investigations depend on subjective rather than objective observations, including partial records, memory, and producer perceptions.[23] Comparisons may be made between the current incidence of disease and a perception of what the rate should be.

In qualitative investigations, causal inferences may be based on the logic of (1) method of agreement, (2) method of difference, or (3) concomitant variations.[20] By the method of agreement, the causal factor is identified when that factor is common to multiple instances of the outcome but other factors are not (eg, discovering outbreaks of toe abscesses among cattle delivered from a particular order buyer in different feedyards). A causal factor might be identified by the method of difference when a particular factor differs but everything else is the same (eg, an outbreak of salmonellosis occurs after 1 feed ingredient in the ration has changed). A causal relationship can be identified by the method of concomitant variations if the likelihood of the outcome changes proportionally, or inversely proportionally, to the level of the proposed risk factor (eg, finding the numbers of polioencephalomalacia cases increasing and decreasing with the sulfur content of feed or water).[20]

When data are available, a quantitative approach may be more powerful for discovering causal relationships, monitoring compliance with recommendations, and evaluating their effectiveness. The best study design for evaluating causal relationships depends on the circumstances. There are 3 basic observational study designs: (1) case-control; (2) cohort or longitudinal; and (3) cross-sectional.

Case-control studies compare odds of exposure among cases with the odds of exposure among noncases. Case-control studies are indicated when the disease is rare and when there are many potential exposures to test. The case-control study design is well suited to many outbreak investigations, especially when the circumstances permit a retrospective comparison of cases (affected subjects) and controls (subjects without the case definition, but otherwise representative of the population). In the author's experience, a common misconception is that controls need to be healthy. However, controls should represent the population of animals the cases come from in every respect except the disease of interest. Therefore, controls may have other illnesses, just not the illness described in the case definition. Attempts to exclude cattle with other diseases from the control definition can be an important source of selection bias.

Cohort and longitudinal studies compare incidence of disease among subjects with an exposure to the incidence of those without the exposure. Cohort and longitudinal studies are indicated when it is possible to follow subjects over time, either prospectively or retrospectively. Cohort and longitudinal studies are observational, meaning that the exposure occurs without assignment. If the exposure can be randomly assigned to individual or groups of cattle (eg, vaccination or not), then, the study design is a randomized controlled trial.[26]

Cross-sectional studies look at the relationship between disease and exposure prevalence at a point in time.[27] The advantage of cross-sectional studies is that they can be completed at a single point in time. However, the relationship lacks any temporal context. That is, cross-sectional studies do not clarify if the exposure or the disease came first. Furthermore, causal exposures or disease incidents that occurred earlier in time may not be measurable at the time of investigation.

Measures of Association

Measures of association are important inferential statistics, because they quantify the strength of the relationship between potential risk factors and the occurrence of disease. When the outcome is dichotomous (eg, diseased or not diseased), the measure of association may be the odds ratio or relative risk, depending on the circumstances. These are comparisons of the odds, probability, or incidence of disease with 1 exposure level compared with another. If the odds ratio or relative risk has a value of 1, then, the exposure is not associated with the disease, because the odds or probability of the disease with the exposure is the same as without. If the odds ratio or relative risk is greater than 1, then, that exposure is positively associated with the disease, because the likelihood of disease is greater when the exposure is present. If the odds ratio or relative risk is less than 1, the exposure is associated with the absence of disease (ie, it is negatively associated with, or protective from, the disease). The further the odds ratio or relative risk is from 1, the stronger the association. Odds ratios are statistically distinct from relative risk, but when the prevalence of disease is rare (eg, <5%), the value of the odds ratio approximates relative risk. Odds ratios are appropriate measures of association for case-control studies, but relative risk is not, because the probability of disease is set by the study design, not the population.

If the outcome is continuous (eg, weight gain), the measure of association is the coefficient of determination, denoted as R^2. The coefficient of determination is an estimate of how well the regression line fits the observed data. It describes how much of the variability in the outcome (the Y variable) is explained by a unit change in the exposure (the X variable). The regression coefficient is the slope of the line. This factor indicates how much a change in the exposure is related to the average of the outcome.[28,29]

Even strong measures of association do not confirm causality. Sometimes, apparent associations are caused by coincidence, confounding, or other sources of bias. Occasionally, the direction of causation is the opposite of what is expected (ie, the outcome was really the cause of the exposure). For example, the investigation may find that use of a particular vaccination protocol (or other management practice) is positively associated with occurrence of the disease. That is, the finding may be that pens of cattle receiving this vaccine were more likely to be sick than cattle in other pens. But, use of the vaccine protocol may have been in response to the perception that those pens of cattle were at greater risk for respiratory disease, rather than the factor leading to higher disease rates.

Significance Testing

Calculators are available online for calculating the odds ratio or relative risk from a 2 x 2 (or 2 x X) contingency table. Many calculators also exist online, or within spreadsheet software, to test the difference in the means of 2 groups (eg, Student's *t* test). These programs report the *P* value to indicate the how likely the outcomes between groups were to have been observed by chance if there really is no effect of the exposure variable. The *P* value is a conditional probability. The probability refers to the likelihood of observing the difference, or greater, in outcomes between the exposure levels. The condition is that the null hypothesis is true, that there is no difference in the effect of the exposure. When the *P* value is small, either a rare event was observed or the null hypothesis is not true. A common convention in science is to reject the null hypothesis when the *P* value is less than or equal to .05.[30] Outbreak investigations are not experimental designs, because sample sizes are often limited by the size of the population or financial resources, and the data may represent a census of the entire population of interest. In an outbreak investigation, the strength of association is more important to causal reasoning than the magnitude of the *P* value. A large *P* value may serve as a caution that the association observed may have occurred by chance, but it should not get in the way of the decision to take action in the face of an outbreak when the strength of evidence suggests that the action is prudent.[17]

CHALLENGES OF OUTBREAK INVESTIGATION IN BEEF CATTLE FEEDLOTS

Investigations of disease or impaired productivity in beef cattle feedyards have unique challenges related to availability of data, various barriers to communication, and the relatively rapid and dynamic temporal and geographic flow of cattle, feed, people, and medications through the system.

Access to Records

It may sometimes be possible to recognize patterns of disease occurrence without data, based on the perceptions of feedlot personnel. However, it becomes increasingly more difficult to relate events to disease outcomes as feedlots become larger and more complex. Feedlot record-keeping systems range from paper-based systems on index cards or in logbooks to elaborate and sophisticated electronic database systems.[31] Most feedlots record health and performance data at the time of treatment or processing, especially in feedlots of larger capacity.[31] Few cattle feeding operations collect animal health data in an easily analyzable format for the purpose of outbreak investigation.

Even sophisticated electronic record-keeping systems may not easily allow cross-referencing of health and performance data. It may be difficult to summarize the number of new cases in the population at risk, calculate the appropriate numerators and denominators of disease incidence, or make associations between risk factors and disease incidence. Usually, if health data are captured in a record-keeping database, the data must be exported to spreadsheet software for analysis. The lack of an easily analyzed health and performance record-keeping system hinders the process of recognizing important hazards, estimating their impact, and making risk management decisions. Some commercially available record-keeping systems are useful for evaluating compliance in the risk management stage, for example, to document treatments and drug withholding times, but not always.

Access to People

Feedyards may have several barriers to communication. Key personnel may know information useful to the investigation but may not be able to speak the same language.

Some employees may be fearful of sharing information. Key personnel may not be forthcoming with information because they are concerned that they will be blamed for the outbreak. It can be challenging to determine if the answers to questions about procedures are factual or if they represent the ideal situation or what the personnel think you might want to hear. If records are available, it may help to cross-reference what is said with what was recorded.

Flow of Animals, Feeds, and People

Feedyards are dynamic systems. Cattle move into and out of feedyards nearly daily. The dynamic population of cattle in feedlots makes describing outbreaks difficult, because the population at risk is constantly changing. Cattle may move from pen to pen within the feedlot, making locational exposures difficult to document. Other portions of feedlots are dynamic, too. Feed rations change and feed ingredients come in and are quickly consumed. Even when a feed intoxication is suspected, it may be difficult to show, because the contaminated feed may have already been fed out. Vaccine lots and other medications also move rapidly through the system. People change jobs or move away, meaning that institutional memory may be short lived. These dynamic factors can make outbreak investigations challenging and show the need for timely collection of records and completing diagnostic testing.

DRAWING CONCLUSIONS FROM AN OUTBREAK INVESTIGATION

The risk management phase begins as soon as the primary facts are in and there is some understanding of the factors associated with the outbreak. This is the phase when decisions are made about how to stop the outbreak. This risk management phase must consider what factors have the most impact on the problem, what it might cost to modify those factors, and what system changes will produce that desired effect.

Measures of Impact

Decisions on risk management of disease should consider the relative importance of various causal factors on those exposed (termed attributable risk of exposure) and on the group (termed population attributable risk).[25]

Not all cases of disease are caused by the factor in question, even when the factor does play a causal role. Attributable risk of exposure estimates the proportion of cases among the exposed that were caused by that exposure.

- Attributable risk of exposure = $(RR - 1)/RR$, where RR is the relative risk of disease caused by that exposure.

An equivalent expression is:

- Attributable risk of exposure = $(I_E - I_{NE})/I_{NE}$, where I_E is the incidence among the exposed and I_{NE} is incidence among the nonexposed

For example, if cattle with black hides were discovered by our investigation to be 3 times more likely to die from heat stress as cattle with lighter hides, the attributable risk of exposure could be calculated as: $(3 - 1)/3 = 2/3$. Two-thirds of the deaths from heat stress in black-hided cattle would be estimated to be caused by their black hides. That statistic means that one-third of the deaths from heat stress in black-hided cattle were caused by some other factor(s). This example helps to show that not all cases among those exposed are caused by the exposure, and helps to quantify how much impact the exposure has on those individuals that have it.

Population attributable risk estimates the burden of disease in the population that is caused by the exposure (risk factor).

- Population attributable risk = $P_E \times (RR - 1)/(P_E \times [RR - 1]) + 1)$, where P_E is the probability of exposure and RR is relative risk of disease because of that exposure.

For example, using the earlier scenario, if 10% of the cattle have black hide, then, 1 of 6 (17%) of the heat stress losses could be attributed to black hides. If 50% of the cattle had black hides, then, 50% of heat stress losses could be attributed to cattle having black hides. If 90% of the cattle in the population have black hides, then, 64% of the heat stress losses could be attributed to black hides. Population attributable risk helps with decisions about what exposures are most important to manage to reduce losses caused by disease or impaired performance. Rare exposures with strong association to disease may not be as important to disease control as common exposures with only moderate association to disease (**Fig. 4**).

Finding the System Solution

The causes of, and solutions to, many outbreaks are inherent to the production system. Understanding the dynamic processes involved in procuring, feeding, and marketing cattle may point to the place in the process at which decisions were made or actions taken that led to the outbreak. Veterinarians who understand system dynamics are uniquely qualified to help their feedlot clients understand how decisions, sometimes far removed from the problem, can affect cattle health and productivity. The challenge is to recognize how the system influences the outcome of concern and find the leverage point for changing the system.

System dynamics is a science for understanding how behaviors in complex systems affect important outcomes.[7] Feedlots are complex adaptive systems: complex, because there are many things going on; adaptive, because the decisions and actions

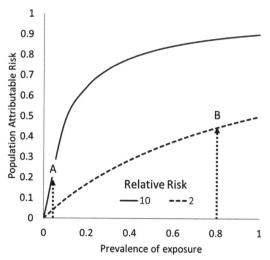

Fig. 4. Comparison of the population attributable risk for exposures with relative risks of 10 and 2 across the range of possible exposure prevalence. Common exposures with less strength of association (*B*) may have greater impact on the health of the population than less common exposures with greater strength of association (*A*).

in the feedlot change in response to what is happening. Because feedlots are complex adaptive systems, it can be difficult to predict what will happen in response to a change in the system. For example, some well-intentioned incentive programs to reward employees for taking certain actions (eg, reporting sick cattle early, hoping that early treatment reduces treatment costs and increases treatment success) have resulted in unexpected outcomes (eg, cattle pulled for treatment unnecessarily and increased treatment costs).

Toe abscesses show the value of systems thinking in the feedyard. Outbreaks of toe abscesses often occur shortly after cattle arrive in the feedlot.[1] Considerable time and effort can be used to treat affected cattle, but the solution to the problem may not come from finding a better treatment or developing a vaccine. The solution may come from evaluating the system of transporting and processing arriving cattle. Toe abscesses are better prevented by understanding that somewhere in the system cattle are wearing down the toe and separating the hoof from the sole by pounding and scraping their toes across hard, abrasive floors.[1] The system solution is to manage how aggressively cattle are moved and the hardness and abrasiveness of the floors on which they are moved.

COMMUNICATING RESULTS
Written Reports

The findings of the outbreak investigation should be reported in writing in a timely fashion that decreases the likelihood of misunderstanding. The report should describe, in simple language, the primary complaint, relevant findings, an interpretation of what factors are contributing to the outbreak, and a succinctly itemized list of the actions needed to solve the problem. Use graphs, charts, and tables to supplement the report. Legal actions may result from the outbreak, so be as complete as possible without overstating the case.

Monitoring Compliance and Resolution

Corrective actions should be measurable so that it is possible to document whether or not the actions were implemented. For example, dates and times that procedures were carried out can be recorded with the initials of the individual completing the task. A record-keeping system should be initiated to monitor compliance and to document whether or not the problem was successfully resolved. A process control approach to recording and analyzing data may identify problems early, before they become costly or harmful to cattle health.[6]

FUTURE CONSIDERATIONS

Few feedyards capture data in a format useful for rapid analysis during an outbreak. The same data useful for investigating outbreaks are likely to be useful for monitoring health and productivity in the absence of a problem. Future feedlot databases need standardized definitions for health and productivity and easy to use calculators for querying, describing, and comparing health events.

SUMMARY

Outbreaks are an unexpected increase in the rate of morbidity, mortality, or impaired productivity. The reasons for investigating outbreaks of disease or impaired productivity are to reduce losses from existing cases, prevent additional cases, and understand how future outbreaks can be avoided. Outbreak investigations are more likely to be successful if an orderly process of investigation is followed using logic based on causal theory. Outbreaks are often the result of decisions and actions taken within the system, even though those actions may have taken place long ago or far away from the current problem. The investigation should be followed up with a clearly written report, which includes recommendations for measurable actions.

REFERENCES

1. Griffin D. Feedlot diseases. Vet Clin North Am Food Anim Pract 1998;14(2): 199–231.
2. Corbin MJ, Griffin D. Assessing performance of feedlot operations using epidemiology. Vet Clin North Am Food Anim Pract 2006;22(1):35–51.
3. Waldner CL, Campbell JR. Disease outbreak investigation in food animal practice. Vet Clin North Am Food Anim Pract 2006;22(1):75–101.
4. Hancock DD, Wikse SE. Investigation planning and data gathering. Vet Clin North Am Food Anim Pract 1988;4:1–15.
5. Smith DR. Field disease diagnostic investigation of neonatal calf diarrhea. Vet Clin North Am Food Anim Pract 2012;28(3):465–81.
6. Reneau JK, Lukas J. Using statistical process control methods to improve herd performance. Vet Clin North Am Food Anim Pract 2006;22(1):171–93.
7. Meadows DH, Wright D. Thinking in systems: a primer. White River Junction (VT): Chelsea Green Pub; 2008.
8. Rothman KJ. Causes. Am J Epidemiol 1976;104:587–92.
9. Duff GC, Galyean ML. Board-invited review: recent advances in management of highly stressed, newly received feedlot cattle. J Anim Sci 2007;85(3):823–40.
10. Popper KR. Science: conjectures and refutations. Conjectures and refutations: the growth of scientific knowledge. 5th edition. New York: Routledge; 1989. p. 33–65.
11. Susser M. Falsification, verification and causal inference in epidemiology: reconsiderations in light of Sir Karl Poppers Philosophy. In: Rothman KJ, editor. Causal inference. 1st edition. Chestnut Hill (MA): Epidemiology Resources Inc; 1988. p. 33–57.
12. Weed DL. Causal criteria and Popperian refutation. In: Rothman KJ, editor. Causal inference. 1st edition. Chestnut Hill (MA): Epidemiology Resources Inc; 1988. p. 15–32.
13. Buck C. Popper's philosophy for epidemiologists. Int J Epidemiol 1975;4:159–68.
14. Rothman KJ. Inferring causal connections–habit, faith or logic?. In: Rothman KJ, editor. Causal inference. 1st edition. Chestnut Hill (MA): Epidemiology Resources Inc; 1988. p. 3–12.
15. Rothman KJ. Causal inference in epidemiology. Modern epidemiology. 1st edition. Boston: Little, Brown and Company; 1986. p. 7–21.
16. Koch R. Die aetiologie der tuberkulose. Mitt Kaiserl Gesundheitsamt 1884;2: 1–88.
17. Hill AB. The environment and disease: association or causation? Proc R Soc Med 1965;58:295–300.
18. Susser M. What is a cause and how do we know one? A grammar for pragmatic epidemiology. Am J Epidemiol 1991;133:635–48.
19. Evans AS. Causation and disease: the Henle-Koch postulates revisited. Yale J Biol Med 1976;49:175–95.
20. Gay JM. Determining cause and effect in herds. Vet Clin North Am Food Anim Pract 2006;22(1):125–47.

21. Mader TL. Feedlot medicine and management. Implants. Vet Clin North Am Food Anim Pract 1998;14(2):279–90.
22. Nagaraja TG, Galyean ML, Cole NA. Nutrition and disease. Vet Clin North Am Food Anim Pract 1998;14(2):257–77.
23. Smith DR. Field epidemiology to manage BRD risk in beef cattle production systems. Anim Health Res Rev 2014;15:180–3.
24. Lessard PR. The characterization of disease outbreaks. Vet Clin North Am Food Anim Pract 1988;4:17–32.
25. Toma B. Dictionary of veterinary epidemiology. 1st English language edition. Ames (IO): Iowa State University Press; 1999.
26. O'Connor AM, Sargeant JM, Gardner IA, et al. The REFLECT statement: methods and processes of creating reporting guidelines for randomized controlled trials for livestock and food safety. Prev Vet Med 2010;93(1):11–8.
27. Shott S. Designing studies that answer questions. J Am Vet Med Assoc 2011; 238(1):55–8.
28. Shott S. Regression. J Am Vet Med Assoc 1991;198:798–801.
29. Shott S. Relationships between more than two variables. J Am Vet Med Assoc 2011;239(5):587–93.
30. Curtis CR, Salman MD, Shott S. P values. J Am Vet Med Assoc 1990;197:318–20.
31. USDA. Feedlot 2011. Part I: Management Practices on U.S. Feedlots with a Capacity of 1,000 or More Head. Fort Collins (CO): USDA–APHIS–VS–CEAH–NAHMS; 2013.

Surgical Management of Common Disorders of Feedlot Calves

Matt D. Miesner, DVM, MS[a],*, David E. Anderson, DVM, MS[b]

KEYWORDS

- Pain • Analgesia • Feedlot • Cattle • Castration • Dehorn • Lameness
- Urethrostomy

KEY POINTS

- Accomplishing necessary procedures involves being efficient, skillful, and aware of methods supporting improvement.
- Procedures causing pain and discomfort are inevitable in feedlot practice and should be balanced with techniques to moderate them.
- Balancing tasks and welfare to provide humanely produced, safe, affordable, and quality consumer products are commissions that the public and animal health professionals share.

INTRODUCTION: NATURE OF THE PROBLEM

Efficiency and cost awareness are highly scrutinized in feedlot practice, as is the product produced. Systemic disease prevention, recognition, and treatment receive the bulk of consideration, with respiratory disease being the most costly disease overall. Shipping and receiving practices are considered critical control points for limiting stress and disease development. Timing of processing procedures relative to arrival time and the association of preventative health measures with feedlot performance receives attention. Castration and dehorning are surgical procedures commonly occurring near arrival processing, whereas other common surgical symptoms affecting musculoskeletal, urogenital, and reproductive systems arise at variable times during the feeding period. All feedlot surgical procedures have indications for intervention and come with a degree of pain and distress inflicted on the animal. Attention should be given to the least painful methods for doing these procedures and applying analgesic techniques to achieve optimal outcome.

The authors have nothing to disclose.
[a] Agricultural Practices, College of Veterinary Medicine, Kansas State University, A-111 Mosier Hall, Manhattan, KS 66506-5802, USA; [b] The University of Tennessee Institute of Agriculture, Veterinary Teaching Hospital, 2407 River Drive, Knoxville, TN 37996, USA
* Corresponding author.
E-mail address: mmiesner@vet.k-state.edu

Vet Clin Food Anim 31 (2015) 407–424
http://dx.doi.org/10.1016/j.cvfa.2015.05.011
0749-0720/15/$ – see front matter Published by Elsevier Inc.

vetfood.theclinics.com

Decision-tree criteria for performing operative procedures should be based on patient signalment (age, size, health status) and sound professional guidance including scientific information when available. Selection of the surgical procedure performed can initially be reduced in number, refined for the sorted class, or eliminated/replaced based on set criteria, thus reducing stress by eliminating total numbers of procedures done. Examples may include tipping horns versus dehorning based on size, not castrating bulls at a certain size or expected short duration in the facility, or eliminating pregnancies in dystocia-prone heifers. Consideration of patient signalment is important, yet should be coupled with facility and operator abilities. When the negative effects of the procedure outweigh the benefits, consider refining the method or eliminating it.

Castration and dehorning effects on performance have been evaluated[1–4] as well as the impact of different methods.[2,5,6] Timing of the procedure, animal performance, and method aside, performing the necessary procedures efficiently and expertly reduces patient distress. Pain exists regardless of skill or method and should be considered and addressed in addition to applying good surgical skills. Analgesic use during these procedures is an important consideration, receiving more and more attention in the public's eye and being evaluated in scientific literature.[7–10] Relatively little data exist looking at analgesic influence on performance parameters in the feedlot,[2,4] but much has been done to evaluate the animals' behavioral response to the procedures themselves.

Major contentions to address are the ability to efficiently and effectively administer analgesia while maintaining a safe and affordable product for human consumption. Cattle feel acute pain, express evidence of delayed and chronic pain, as well as demonstrate pathologic pain that becomes unresponsive to traditional analgesics and application methods. The pain pathway can be addressed at the forefront through preemptive pain management by supplying analgesics locally or systemically before stimulation. Local anesthetics eliminate the acute sting but only interrupt the resulting delayed discomfort. Operators should be trained in various methods of local/regional application of analgesia, as some regional techniques are more efficiently and effectively applied than direct infusion in the surgical site.[11] Local anesthetics have to be properly applied/injected but also a short delay in effect recognized.[4] Delay in analgesic effect of only seconds to a couple minutes greatly reduces processing speed when looked at solely; however, patient cooperation may offset that time significantly, especially with less adequate physical restraint. Preemptive use of nonsteroidal anti-inflammatory drugs (NSAIDs) may suppress delayed pain from the acute procedure.[12] Methods to provide systemic analgesia can be applied in many situations quite effectively, affordably, and safely.[13] Although no drugs are specifically labeled for analgesia in the United States, extralabel drug use guidelines are valid while the operator targets the physiologic pathways of providing analgesia.[13]

THERAPEUTIC OPTIONS AND/OR SURGICAL TECHNIQUES
Castration

Castration is likely the most common surgery performed in feedlot medicine. Strong efforts should be made to assure castration of young bull calves occur as close to calving and weaning as possible to limit complications with castrating larger bulls. Regardless of efforts, some cow-calf operations will not be able to castrate before feedlot arrival. Methods of castration (orchiectomy) can be surgical or performed with various nonsurgical techniques, sometimes referred to as bloodless methods. Bloodless methods induce ischemic necrosis of the testicles and/or scrotum. Banding methods remove the scrotum and testes, whereas Burdizzo emasculatome will disrupt the testicular cord resulting in testicular atrophy yet scrotal retention. Surgical castration methods have 3 goals: open the scrotum to remove both testicles, provide adequate hemostasis, and leave the scrotum open sufficiently for drainage. Benefits, contraindications, and complications exist for all methods of castration. Patient signalment and history, operator training, and working facility should all factor into choosing castration methods if they are to be undertaken at all.

Standing castrations with cattle restrained in a squeeze chute are by far the most common restraint method. Recumbency may be required when testicles are positioned high in the inguinal region with cryptorchids or cattle that have incomplete castrations (ie, missed testicles) from previous attempts before arrival. Working facilities vary considerably and should be evaluated and refined for the types of cattle being worked and available resources, including physical labor. Limited stress handling and enhanced worker safety are initial goals toward successful procedure outcomes.

Some direct preparation is necessary before castration. Removal of gross organic contaminants and implementing cursory antiseptic cleansing is strongly recommended. Tetanus is a real complication risk of castration and should be anticipated to be more likely with gross contamination of organic debris favoring *Clostridium tetani* organisms and castration methods resulting from scrotal necrosis.[14] Cleansing solutions in open containers should be changed regularly or closed delivery systems, such as handheld sprayers, can be used to provide reliably clean solutions. Vaccine status against *C tetani* should be up to date, and boosting with a tetanus toxoid at the time of castration may help limit cases. Clinical tetanus takes longer to develop than the effective duration of tetanus antitoxin; therefore, parenteral tetanus antitoxin would not provide adequate protection.

After cleansing, inject 3 to 5 mL of 2% lidocaine over each testicular cord in the neck of the scrotum as well as in between the testicles to anesthetize the median raphe, effectively blocking the testicular structures and scrotum. Expect 2 to 5 minutes for the anesthetic to take effect. An additional 10 to 15 mL of lidocaine injected into the parenchyma of each testicle of bulls with more than 500 lb body weight (BW) can be considered.[15] A topical anesthetic gel product (Tri-Solfen) has been investigated in Australia indicating beneficial pain alleviation during surgical castration of 3- to 4-month-old calves.[9]

Caudal epidural anesthesia has been evaluated with mixed levels of effectiveness for castration.[16–19] Currently, it is best used as a portion of a multimodal component but limited as a lone technique. The primary limitation with epidural anesthesia is placing the anesthetic cranial enough to block all branches supplying sensory input to the testicles without also anesthetizing the motor support nerves of the pelvic limbs. Anesthetics of consideration are 2% lidocaine or alpha-2 drugs, such as xylazine.[19] Lidocaine anesthetizes both motor and sensory nerves and must be given at a high enough volume to block all the nerves supplying the testicle originating from the lumbar region to be effective in castration. There is a fine line regarding nerves providing testicular sensation and those of pelvic limb support in the spinal cord. Higher volumes of lidocaine can possibly result in recumbency as it travels cranial to block the major motor nerves to the pelvic limbs.

Xylazine induces a mixed sensory and motor blockade, weighs heavier on sensory than motor nerves, and can be diluted and given at higher volumes to reach the testicular origin branches with less risk of recumbency.[19] Once absorbed from the epidural space, xylazine also provides some systemic analgesia and minor sedation. A major limitation of xylazine epidural use is that the time to effect takes 30 to 45 minutes. Xylazine exerts a longer local analgesic effect than lidocaine that may be beneficial in suppressing chronic pain. Systemic NSAIDs are effective at providing analgesia for the delayed or chronic pain that results postoperatively.[20] Performing these methods of analgesia, although not practical in every procedure, should be recognized and used based on individual patient expectations for intraoperative responses and postoperative recovery.

Surgical castration involves opening the scrotum to gain access to the testicles. This procedure is done by sharply removing the distal half of the scrotum with a scalpel, making 2 separate longitudinal skin incisions over each with a scalpel, or using a Newberry knife to create the scrotal opening. The most efficient use of the Newberry knife is to orient the blade to cut through the lateral sides of the scrotum and median raphe in one pulling motion, exposing both testicles for removal. Whichever method is used to open the scrotum, the resulting opening after castration should be sufficient to promote good postsurgical drainage. The testicles should be visible after the scrotal incision is made. Before making the incision, the scrotum should be evaluated and palpated for asymmetry to predict preexisting problems, such as an inguinal hernia.

To remove the testicles, gain exposure to the proximal testicular cord before severing it in a controlled manner while providing sufficient hemostasis. Most castrations are done using a closed technique whereby the tunica vaginalis is not opened. Grasp the testicle and retract, removing the surrounding fascia and possibly the cremaster attachment to expose the spermatic cord sufficiently for hemostasis application by crushing (emasculator application), ligating, or twisting the cord before transection and removal of the testicle. Most feedlot bulls will require some method of hemostasis to reduce the risk of fatal hemorrhage caused by the size, beyond simply pulling testicles as can be done in neonatal and preweaned calves. Emasculator instruments of various configurations are available to crush and sever the cord. The emasculator type should be sufficient for the size of the testicular cord being applied to, and emasculators should be inspected and serviced or replaced as the crushing and cutting surfaces wear. A Henderson tool (Stone Manufacturing, Kansas City, MO) can be used to twist the cord until rupture providing hemostasis; however, it should be used properly to avoid scrotal contamination. Absorbable ligature material should be used if this method is chosen for hemostasis. Surgical castration can be done in very large bulls with proper restraint and technique; however, increased operative and postoperative complications can be expected the larger the bull.

Bloodless castration methods depend on disruption of the blood supply to the testicles without opening the scrotum. Various-sized bands and banding devices suited for the size of scrotum are available. Small rubber elastrator bands are unlikely to be sufficient in feedlot bulls. Larger banding devices, such as the Callicrate system (No-Bull Enterprises LLC, St Francis, KS) or California Bander (InoSol Co LLC, El Centro, CA), are better suited for larger bulls. Ischemic necrosis of the scrotum and testicles is expected to take at least 10 days and up to 3 weeks to complete. Although sharp surgical pain is not expected with band application, delayed pain and discomfort are evident during the time the process is occurring.[2,4] In addition, the tissue environment surrounding the band is welcoming of trapped clostridial organisms; therefore, proper cleansing and preventive measures against tetanus should be part of the process. The operator must be sure to have trapped both testicles is the scrotum and not applied the band too proximal possibly affecting the penis.

Application of a Burdizzo emasculatome is an alternative to banding whereby each cord is palpated through the neck of the scrotum, positioned to the lateral aspect of the neck away from the median raphe, and crushed with the instrument for 10 to 30 seconds and released. Manually stretching/disrupting the testicular cord while the instrument is applied can be done. The operator should do both sides separately

(2 applications) and offset the level of application proximal or distal by a few centimeters. The intension here is to disrupt the testicular blood supply and maintain the scrotum by avoiding the scrotal blood supply in the median raphe. Anaerobic conditions will still be present inviting tetanus risk, and operators must be sure to have isolated each cord properly.

Postcastration complications and management

Hemorrhage after surgical castration is expected but can be excessive if inadequate hemostasis was achieved and can be fatal. Clinical signs of excessive blood loss that indicate intervention include depression, increased heart rate and respiratory rate, weakness and ataxia, and possibly uncoordinated aggression caused by hypoxia. Attempting to find and isolate severed blood vessels after castration is difficult and often unrewarding because of retraction of the vessels far proximal to the resected scrotum. However, if one is to pursue the task, identify the most secure method of restraint providing the most visual inspection, which may require placing the animal in recumbency. Make sure the operator's hands are clean or gloved, and try to be systematic in identifying the primary source of the bleeding. If the source in not evident, consider packing the scrotum with gauze (kaolin impregnated if available) and compressing with adherent bandage material wrapped tightly around the scrotum.

It can also be fairly straightforward to collect blood from a healthy donor (10 mL/kg BW) and transfuse it into anemic patients to provide some support and clotting factors. For example, a 700-lb steer can safely provide 3L ($\sim$10 mL/kg) of blood. Clinically anemic patients of similar size may need twice that for short-term stability for recovery. There are no standards for crossmatching in cattle, and reaction is highly unlikely because of blood type variations. Practical used collection containers and recipes for anticoagulants in cattle practice are described.[21] A simple method is to combine 20 g of powdered sodium citrate per 1 gallon of collected whole blood.

Inflammation is expected after castration, tending to peak during the first 2 to 5 days after surgery. Although NSAIDs may provide analgesic benefit after castration, overall inflammation during healing may not be reduced compared with the cattle not receiving NSAIDs at castration.[22] Inflammation and healing after surgical castration is expected to take on average between 3 and 4 weeks. Contamination is expected; however, infection should be recognized early and treated.

Dehorning

Dehorning will be done in the squeeze chute and possibly at the time of castration if both are indicated. Stress induced by castration and dehorning at the same time does not seem to be additive based on one study as long as analgesics are administered before performing the tasks together.[23] Dehorning is the act of removing the entire horn, which is in contrast to tipping that is regarded as partial removal of the less vascular and innervated distal end of the horn. Both practices have the goal of improving animal and worker safety, reducing carcass damage, and facilitating animal movement and handling. Horn tipping may provide some benefits toward safety and handling but does not tend to result in less carcass damage.[24]

Overall growth of horn during the feeding period may be minimal in some animals, and consideration of forgoing dehorning or tipping horns of short length on arrival should be considered. Horn tipping still carries the risk of infection as contaminants may ascend through the small exposed vascular and cornual tracts to the sinuses resulting in frontal sinusitis or local infections; however, it is regarded as less invasive and painful than dehorning. Banding methods have been shown to induce major discomfort and have a high failure rate in cattle.[25] Proper dehorning involves the removal of the cornual epithelium and stopping the vascular supply at the base of the horn.

Manually restrain the head and neck in and squeeze the chute. The cornual nerve supply can be targeted for anesthesia by palpating the frontal crest of the skull midway between the lateral canthus of the eye and the base of the horn. Deposit 10 to 15 mL of 2% lidocaine subcutaneously there to block the cornual nerve (**Fig. 1**). Cranial cervical sensory nerve branches become more substantial in larger horns, supplying sensation to the caudal horn; therefore, an additional 5 to 10 mL of lidocaine should be infused at the caudal horn base as well. The horn can be removed at its base with sufficient manual or automatic dehorning tools that scoop or guillotine the base from its attachment to the skull. The major blood supply can usually be visualized at the ventral base of the resulting wound. Hemostasis is achieved by pulling or twisting the vessel with a hemostatic clamp. Frequently, the frontal sinus is exposed in larger horns, possibly leading to frontal sinusitis as a complication. When the situation allows, consider surgical dehorning to allow closure of the skin over the dehorning wound and frontal sinus.[26] Tipping of horns can also result in frontal sinusitis caused by ascending infection through the horn tubules and vascular channels.

Enucleation

Trauma, infection, or retrobulbar lymphadenopathy may cause damage to the eyes of feedlot calves sufficient to justify enucleation. Field surgery is a viable option for elimination of pain, source of infection, and return to productivity. Although the surgical techniques are not new, thorough physical examination, proper preparation of patients, appropriate perioperative management, and good surgical technique will assure the best results possible.

Sedation is warranted in most feedlot calves to facilitate efficient enucleation. The author most often uses a combination of xylazine (0.05 mg/kg BW intramuscularly [IM]), butorphanol (0.02 mg/kg IM), and ketamine (0.1 mg/kg IM) for standing restraint. The addition of dissociative doses of ketamine aids in the management of fractious patients, and these 3 drugs in combination have been referred to as a K-Stun technique.

Ocular nerve blocks often include motor blockade of the eyelids and sensory and motor nerve blockade of the ophthalmic nerve. Surgical manipulation of the eye is facilitated by nerve blockade of the eyelids. An auriculopalpebral nerve block can

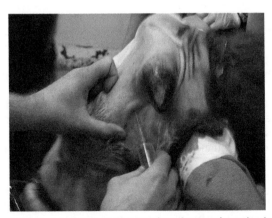

Fig. 1. The cornual nerve can be located cranial and ventral to the horn overlying the palpable facial crest.

be placed to reduce upper eyelid movement before performing a retrobulbar block. The auriculopalpebral nerve can be palpated as it crosses the zygomatic arch, roughly 5 to 6 cm behind the supraorbital process. Inject 5 mL of 2% lidocaine hydrochloride subcutaneously on the dorsal aspect of the zygomatic arch at this location. The 4-point retrobulbar block is technically easier and can be done more rapidly as compared with the Peterson eye block. In this technique, an 18-gauge, 7.5-cm (3.5-in) long needle is introduced through the skin on the dorsal, lateral, ventral, and medial aspects of the eye, at 12-, 3-, 6-, and 9-o'clock positions, respectively. The needle is directed behind the globe using the bony orbit as a guide. When the needle is introduced into retrobulbar sheath, the eye will move slightly with the tug of the needle. After this location is reached and aspiration is performed to assure that the needle is not in a vessel, 5 to 10 mL of lidocaine (2%) is deposited at each site. Mydriasis indicates a successful block.

Infection of the surgical site is one of the most common complications of ocular surgery when done in field settings. Care must be taken to reduce the risk of contamination to the planned surgical site. The hair should be clipped and the skin disinfected with solutions, such as povidone-iodine (Betadine) or chlorhexidine. The ear should be retracted and draped and the lateral portion of the halter covered to decrease contamination to the surgical site. Saline rinse rather than alcohol should be used between the disinfectant scrubs to prevent painful irritation to the cornea.

A transpalpebral ablation technique is used to remove the eye. The upper and lower eyelids are sutured closed; alternatively, eyelids can be closed using multiple towel clamps. A circumferential skin incision is made approximately 1 cm from the edges of the eyelids. Using a combination of blunt and sharp dissection, Mayo scissors are used to dissect through the orbicularis oculi muscle, fascia, and subcutaneous tissue surrounding the eye. The interior of the bony orbit is used as a guide. The medial and lateral canthal ligaments are sharply transected to allow access to the caudal aspect of the orbit. As there is a large vessel associated with the medial canthus, transection of the medial canthal ligaments is best left until necessary. The retrobulbar musculature and the optic nerve sheath should be transected as far caudally as feasible. A vascular clamp can aid in hemostasis while additional excision of the remaining orbital tissue is undertaken. The skin incision can be closed with a nonabsorbable suture, such as No. 3 nylon, in a simple, continuous, forward, interlocking or interrupted horizontal mattress pattern. The skin sutures are removed routinely in 14 to 21 days.

Enucleation postoperative care

The animal should be kept in a sick pen for several days after surgery to allow for swelling and inflammation to subside. Daily observation of the surgical site and assessment of general well-being is recommended until suture removal. Postoperative complications can include simple incisional infection, orbital infections, dehiscence of the suture, or significant infections of the periorbital tissue. Cattle often demonstrate pruritus after surgery, which can lead to incisional dehiscence caused by head rubbing. If purulent drainage is noted during the course of healing in an enucleation procedure, the sutures can be removed and the cavity flushed with a dilute disinfectant solution daily until resolution of the orbital infection. Antibiotic therapy and antiinflammatory therapy are recommended for 5 days after surgery.

Tracheostomy

Tracheotomy provides emergency airway access in patients with upper airway obstruction.[27] In cattle, bacterial infection is the most common cause of obstruction of the pharynx and larynx. Calf diphtheria may be the most common cause of chronic obstructive breathing because of granulation tissue and adhesions (honker calves). Laryngeal necrobacillosis (calf diphtheria) refers to infection of the larynx and pharynx with *Fusobacterium necrophorum*. However, laryngitis may also be associated with laryngeal ulceration and infection with *Pasteurella* spp, *Haemophilus* spp, and *Mycoplasma* spp.[28] Infection is established when the bacteria gain access to submucosal tissues through abrasions or disruption of the overlying mucosae. Infectious bovine rhinotracheitis virus infection should be suspected when extensive laryngotracheitis and pseudomembrane formation is found. Swelling and inflammation result in diminished glottic diameter and cause respiratory distress. Double-muscled calves affected with necrotic laryngitis were found to have increased total pulmonary resistance and decreased dynamic lung compliance and arterial oxygen tension.[29]

When laryngeal swelling causes severe limitations of airflow, a temporary tracheostomy will allow relatively normal breathing so that medical treatment of the infection can be done. Ideally, antibiotic selection is based on bacterial culture and sensitivity results; but empirical antibiotic therapy may be curative.[30] In one report, cattle having septic laryngitis in which the infection had failed to respond to antibiotics were treated by surgical debridement via laryngotomy.[31] Twenty-three calves and adult cattle were treated surgically by laryngotomy, and this treatment resulted in a 74% success rate. General anesthesia was administered via a tracheal tube placed through a temporary tracheostomy. A ventral midline laryngotomy was made by incising the thyroid, cricoid, and cranial tracheal cartilages.

Arytenoid chondritis is rarely diagnosed but is not uncommonly seen in cattle affected with necrotic laryngitis. Arytenoid swelling may cause inspiratory dyspnea and respiratory noise (honker calves). The narrowed glottis causes increased airway turbulence that may cause the arytenoid swelling to persist. Medical treatment (antibiotics and antiinflammatory drugs) is usually curative. Administration of steroids is indicated when acute swelling with severe dyspnea is found. Temporary tracheostomy can be used as palliative therapy in calves when chronic arytenoid swelling caused sufficient inspiratory dyspnea to limit activity and feed intake. Partial or subtotal arytenoidectomy via a laryngotomy is only indicated when necrosis of the arytenoid cartilage is found.[32] Scar-tissue formation causing reduced glottic diameter (webbing) may require ventral laryngotomy and surgical reduction of the scar tissue.[31]

Excessive scar tissue is usually formed on the vocal cords (vocal process of the arytenoid cartilage); excessive granulation is usually formed on the medial aspect of the arytenoid cartilages. For debridement of the larynx and removal of necrotic cartilage, a ventral midline incision centered over the larynx is made; the sternohyoideus muscles are separated; and the thyroid cartilage, cricothyroid ligament, cricoid cartilage, and the first 2 tracheal rings are incised.[33] Volkmann retractors are helpful to expose the larynx. Necrotic tissues are debrided and excised. The laryngotomy may be closed primarily, partially closed with implantation of a Penrose drain, or left open for second intention healing. A tracheostomy may be required for intubation of the trachea when general anesthesia is used, and the tracheostomy should be maintained after surgery until laryngeal swelling has diminished sufficiently for adequate breathing.

Laryngeal granuloma may be formed as a result of trauma to the arytenoid cartilage or vocal cords (rough feeds, balling gun, orogastric tube), infection (necrotic laryngitis), infectious bovine rhinotracheitis, laryngeal ulcers,[28] and foreign bodies.[34] Differential diagnoses should include laryngeal abscess, hematoma, neoplasia, and papilloma. When inspiratory dyspnea is present, surgical removal of the granulation tissue is indicated; a temporary tracheostomy may be needed during the healing period.

Temporary tracheostomy is readily performed in field settings and is clinically useful for defined periods of time (<30 days). When a long-term airway is needed, a permanent tracheostomy may be indicated. Sedation is not routinely used to avoid cardiorespiratory collapse of an animal already dyspneic. When needed, sedation using butorphanol (0.05 mg/kg intravenously) offers a safer alternative to xylazine. In an emergency situation, the surgery site is not aseptically prepared. However, whenever possible, the ventral part of the neck is clipped and aseptically prepared. A line block is performed on the ventral midline at the junction of the cranial and middle third of the neck using 10 mL of 2% lidocaine. The location of the surgery site is important; if done too low on the neck, more dissection is needed because the trachea is located deeper beneath the skin. Preoperative preparation is best done with the head in a relaxed position. At the time of surgery, the head is elevated to expose the ventral neck to the surgeon.

Grasp the trachea with the middle and index fingers. A sharp surgical incision in made through the skin directly on the midline over the trachea using the No. 10 scalpel blade. Make the skin incision 5 to 10 cm long depending on the patients' size. Next, make the best attempts to separate the paired sternohyoideus and sternothyroideus muscles along their median raphe. Make sure the incision is long enough to visualize several tracheal rings to facilitate manipulation and incision between the rings.

Grasp the trachea and make a sharp stab incision between 2 tracheal rings through the annular ligament and tracheal mucosa. Extend the tracheal incision far enough to place a tracheostomy tube, but avoid incising more than one-half the circumference of the trachea. Overaggressive tracheal incisions may result in tracheal collapse after healing.

Place a tracheostomy tube through the incision after temporarily widening the opening between the tracheal rings using tissue forceps or towel clamps. Several types of tracheostomy tubes are available for large animals. Self-retaining, stainless steel split tubes are ideal because they are easily inserted, have a low risk of tracheal obstructions, are easily cleaned, and can be repeatedly used. The tube should then be secured in place by suturing it to the skin (**Fig. 2**). Suture the skin dorsal and ventral to the tracheotomy site with a nonabsorbable monofilament suture in an interrupted or cruciate pattern so that dislodgement is prevented. A petrolatum-based ointment applied around the tracheotomy site after completing the procedure will help keep the surgery site free from mucus and debris.

Complications of tracheostomy may include localized infection, pneumonia, and tracheal stenosis. Exuberant granulation may develop during healing. Subcutaneous emphysema, tracheal mucosa undermining, septic fasciitis, and tracheal collapse may develop occasionally. Monitor closely for a sudden increase in respiratory difficulty. Ideally, the tracheal tube and tracheotomy site should be cleaned twice daily; mucus buildup on the tube should be evaluated, possibly indicating more frequent cleaning. Systemic antimicrobials should be started at the time of the procedure and continued 5 to 7 days after removal of the tube.

Tongue Amputation

Direct tongue trauma, penetrating and encircling foreign bodies, and primary infection occur on occasion in cattle. Excessive salivation, anorexia, foul breath, and persistent protrusion of the tongue indicate oropharyngeal disease. Oral inspection may reveal a variety of oral lesions, including ulceration and vesicles that should be closely evaluated for the possibility of foreign animal disease, reportable vesicular diseases, or evidence of systemic disease whereby tongue amputation will not benefit the animal (eg, bovine viral diarrhea virus). Most lacerations can heal with cleansing and

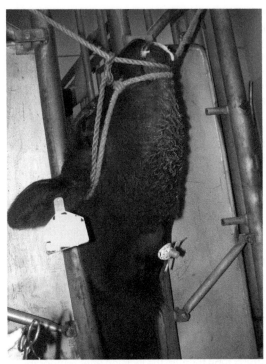

Fig. 2. Angus calf immediately following placement of tracheostomy tube. Calf is restrained in a head gate with the head extended upwards to facilitate access to the proximal one-third of the neck.

supportive care, and foreign bodies can be removed without the need for surgical amputation. However, these conditions can cause an inability of the calf to retract the tongue into the oral cavity, resulting in ongoing trauma and preventing feed consumption (**Fig. 3**). Cattle can retain the ability to drink and consume feed with tongue amputation.

Amputation of the tongue should be limited to the portion rostral to the frenulum. Sedation with xylazine to achieve recumbency is desired, followed by local anesthetic infusion of 2% lidocaine in the base of the tongue and sublingual. An oral speculum will facilitate visualization and exposure. A long forceps or similar instrument positioned just cranial to the frenulum facilitates a straight and controlled incisional amputation (**Fig. 4**). Alternatively, surgical tubing, Penrose drain, or length of rolled gauze can be wrapped caudal to the portion of tongue to be amputated, both for traction and hemostasis. A sharp excision is made, such that the dorsal and ventral aspects taper caudoventral or caudodorsal, respectively, to the center of the tongue (see **Fig. 4**). This technique allows the dorsal and ventral tongue to be opposed with soft, braided suture material, preferably an absorbable suture. Postoperative antiinflammatories and antibiotics are indicated, and rapid healing is expected to occur. Recheck the surgery site in 1 week, and remove the sutures if needed.

Perineal Urethrostomy

Feedlot steers are at an increased risk of urethral obstruction by urinary calculi caused by consuming calculogenic diets and urethral anatomy. Early clinical signs of obstruction are mild to moderate colic with pacing, flagging the tail, and kicking at the

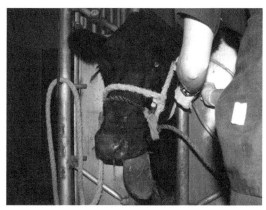

Fig. 3. Injury may prevent retraction of the tongue within the oral cavity, and amputation may be indicated.

abdomen predominating. Initial clinical signs can be missed, and subsequent clinical signs caused by rupture of the bladder (ascites) or urethra (ventral subcutaneous swelling) may be recognized. Both conditions may be accompanied with mixed degrees of depression caused by uremia. Cattle have a great ability to tolerate uremia through metabolic pathways, thus masking a ruptured bladder for days with only increasing signs of depression and decreased feed intake.[35,36] Although urethral rupture and ventral swelling are quite obvious, bladder rupture can be mistaken for other common feedlot diseases. A full physical examination including inspecting a dry preputial orifice, ballottement of a fluid filled abdomen, and uremic breath are all strongly suggestive of proximal urinary obstruction and rupture. Once urethral obstruction is diagnosed, redirecting the urethra opening proximal to the obstruction should be undertaken through urethrostomy.

The most common portion of the urethra where the obstruction occurs is at the level of the distal sigmoid flexure and should be palpated during the physical examination

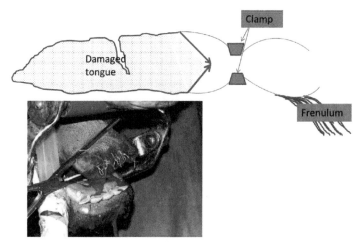

Fig. 4. Diagram of the tongue from the lateral side indicating the orientation of the excision (*red arrows*) toward the center. The dorsal and ventral halves are then sutured together as seen in the photograph.

for signs of increased pain. A urethrostomy should be approached at some level from the distal sigmoid flexure and proximal to the ischial arch. The penis is more movable at the level of the sigmoid but strongly connected with tissues more proximal near the ischium. The most common approach is either over the sigmoid flexure or within about 20 cm of the ischium distal. These areas allow the urethra to be positioned and fixed to the surface of the skin under little tension. The area of the surgical approach should be clipped and prepped for surgery. A combination of local infiltration and caudal epidural with 2% lidocaine are used for anesthesia. A sharp skin incision is made parallel with the penis, and the soft tissues are bluntly dissected until the penis is isolated and easily retracted to the skin incision. A urethrotomy can be performed sharply with a scalpel. Occasionally, urethral calculi are identified and removed at the urethrotomy site (most common at the sigmoid location). A polypropylene catheter can be inserted into the urethra followed by lavage with saline. A urethrostomy can be performed by first anchoring the penis to the skin and subcutaneous tissue with mattress suture through the tunica albuginea and corpus spongiosum penis, followed by opposing the urethral mucosa with the skin.

An alternative to urethrostomy is a penile transection and transposition surgery whereby the penis is transected and the proximal portion redirected and fixed outwardly under little tension by suturing the skin to the tunica albuginea of the penis (**Figs. 5** and **6**). The dorsal penile artery should be identified and ligated. Significant hemorrhage is expected with the exposed corpus spongiosum penis and should be controlled through ligation and compression. The exposed stump can also be hollowed with a partial wedge in the corpus spongiosum, and the edges are sutured together. When there is extensive subcutaneous urine accumulation, the surgeon may choose to remove the distal penis from the sheath by caudal traction through the approach before transecting it. Penectomy by this means may enhance drainage from the subcutaneous tissues but is not considered necessary in all cases by this author.

Complications and management

Significant urethritis and inflammation proximal to the chosen urethrostomy site may be present, resulting in failure of the urethrostomy. Attempts at catheterization of

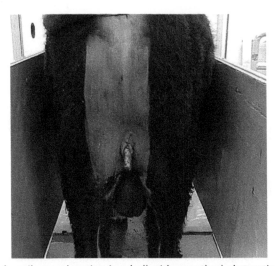

Fig. 5. Completed penile translocation in a bull with a urethral obstruction. This procedure was done at the distal location near the sigmoid flexure.

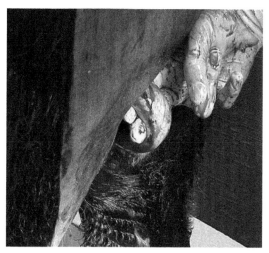

Fig. 6. The penis has been isolated and exposed. At this point, a urethrotomy, urethrostomy, or penile translocation can be completed.

the bladder are often unrewarding because of the presence of the urethral diverticulum at the ischial arch.[37] Very proximal urethrostomy may allow passage of a urinary catheter into the bladder by straightening the proximal penis and providing an open route to the bladder. Aside from local infection and hemorrhage, a common postoperative complication is stricture at the urethrostomy site.[37]

Rumenotomy and Rumenostomy

Rumen surgery may be performed in feedlot cattle for a variety of reasons, including traumatic reticuloperitonitis (hardware disease), ruminal foreign bodies, frothy boat, acute free gas bloat, chronic bloat, recurrent bloat, grain overload, and toxin ingestion.[38–41] Rumenotomy is useful for removal of rumen contents or foreign bodies; rumenostomy is more often performed for the management of bloat and rumen dietary adaptive problems.

Rumenotomy involves making a left paralumbar fossa laparotomy incision through the skin; the external, internal, and transverse abdominal muscles; and followed by the peritoneum. A grid approach may be used by splitting the fibers of the abdominal muscles parallel to their direction.[38,39] The dorsal sac of the rumen is then exteriorized and secured before creation of the rumenotomy incision. The dorsal sac of the rumen can be secured to the skin using towel clamps or sutures in a continuous inverting suture pattern, such as a Connell or a Cushing (**Fig. 7**). A variety of devices have been described as a means of exteriorizing and stabilizing the rumen quickly and efficiently.

Several devices have been developed to anchor the rumen following exteriorization and speed up the rumenotomy procedure.[42] These devices have a hole in the center of a board or ring through which the dorsal sac of the rumen is pulled through. A series of hooks placed through the cut edge of the rumen attach the rumenotomy incision to the board. The board helps to decrease abdominal contamination but limits the accessibility of the rumen.[40] At best, rumen surgery is considered a clean contaminated surgery because an intestinal viscera is penetrated. Antibiotics and antiinflammatory drugs are essential to provide the best chance to prevent peritonitis associated with the procedure.[42] The complication rate associated with rumen surgery is expected to be low when contamination of the abdomen can be avoided. The prognosis and

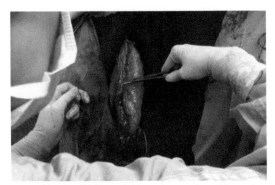

Fig. 7. The rumen has been sutured to the skin by suturing the seromuscular layer of the rumen to the external surface of the skin, creating a tight seal so as to prevent contamination of the abdominal muscles or peritoneum with rumen fluid when the rumenotomy incision is made. The rumenotomy incision is being sutured in this image with a 2-Cushing pattern.

outcome largely depend on the presenting complaint and preoperative condition of the animal and not operative factors.

Rumenostomy is an excellent tool for the management of chronic bloat and administration of therapeutic products and nutritional supplements in calves with rumen dysfunction or maladaptation. Rumenostomy is done similarly to rumenotomy except that a much more discrete incision is made. The location of the rumenostomy should be positioned such that the dorsal sac of the rumen is entered in the free gas portion. As a rule of thumb, an imaginary line can be drawn from the caudal most point of the costochondral arch of the last rib to the point of the tuber coxae. The free gas portion of the dorsal sac of the rumen should be dorsal to a horizontal line drawn through the midpoint of this line. In calves, this point is often 1 handsbreadth caudal to the last rib and 1 handsbreadth ventral to the third lumbar vertebrae. A 5-cm circular portion of skin is removed, and blunt dissection is used to separate the muscle fibers parallel to their orientation (grid approach) until the peritoneal cavity is penetrated. Then, the dorsal sac of the rumen is grasped and exteriorized. The rumen is incised, and the cut edge is sutured to the skin using nonabsorbable suture material placed using either interrupted or continuous suture patterns. These stomas are useful for prolonged management of rumen dysfunction as they are not likely to heal closed. Alternatively, the seromuscular wall of the rumen can be sutured to the skin edge, and a circular portion of the rumen wall can be excised (**Fig. 8**). This type of rumenostomy will often heal in 2 to 6 weeks as the free cut edge of the rumen contracts.

Midline Cesarean Section

Pregnant heifers not only present a financial risk based on performance and yield data but also dystocia risks.[43] Frequently, the heifer's pelvis will be unable to accommodate natural parturition. Excessive traction with a calf jack can result in a down heifer and other welfare issues. Cesarean section could be an option in some instances. Standing flank cesarean, although common in cow-calf practice, may have pitfalls in feedlot heifers because of poorly accommodating chutes, heifer cooperation, undesirable muscle trauma, and possibly a dead fetus with higher risk of catastrophic peritonitis. A midline cesarean section can be performed quickly, using controlled rope restraint and sedation, and improve uterine exposure to remove dead fetuses without abdominal contamination.

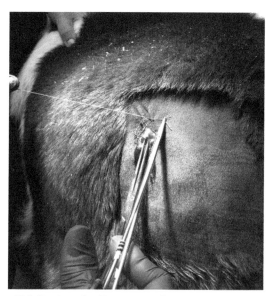

Fig. 8. Limousine calf following the first stage of a temporary rumenostomy. A circular portion of the skin has been excised, the abdominal muscles separated using a grid technique, and the seromuscular wall of the rumen sutured to the skin. Following this procedure, the rumen wall can be incised or a circular segment excised to provide relief of rumen distention.

Preemptive broad-spectrum antimicrobials and NSAIDs are indicated to limit postoperative infection and pain. A high-volume caudal epidural with 2% lidocaine and/or alpha-2 drug can be considered in these cases to reduce kicking during the surgery as well as provide some surgical anesthesia. Pelvic limb ataxia can be expected to persist for a few hours after onset; therefore, the heifer should have good footing. Consider applying hobbles postoperatively. Rope restraints should be applied to help cast the heifer and hold her in position. The ventral midline should be generously clipped from flank fold to flank fold and sternum to udder, followed by a sterile scrub and subcutaneous lidocaine infiltration.

Incise the skin and subcutaneous tissues on midline and identify the linea alba. Incise the linea alba with a scalpel blade 20 to 30 cm. The omental sling of the omentum will likely be identified first on entering the abdomen unless the uterus is outside the sling. If the omentum is encountered, reach through the incision and caudal toward the pelvic brim until the caudal extent of the omental sling is palpated. Grasp the caudal extent of the sling and pull it cranial like a curtain until the uterus is exposed. Expose the uterus through the incision by grasping a limb or head or cradling the uterine horn through the incision. Incise the uterus and remove the calf while keeping the uterus outside the abdomen, which is very important when the fetus is dead or emphysematous.

Suture the uterus in an inverting pattern with absorbable suture material. The author prefers a No. 3 chromic gut using a 2-layer Cushing or Utrecht pattern. The linea alba provides very strong and identifiable tissue for closure. Close the linea alba using absorbable suture material with strong tensile strength in an interrupted or continuous interrupted pattern. A nonabsorbable suture has a greater risk of providing a nidus for persistent infection resulting in chronic wound drainage and failure of repair. A sufficient suture example would be a No. 3 polyglactin 910 (Ethicon Inc, Somerville, NJ) using a cruciate or inverted cruciate pattern. In horses, a continuous pattern was shown to be superior to interrupted patterns as far as bursting strength at the linea alba.[44] A continuous layer of absorbable sutures can be used to close the subcutaneous tissue and dead space. Finally, the skin is closed in a Ford interlocking pattern. The run of skin sutures can be interrupted at some point to avoid losing the entire line if drainage is needed postoperatively.

SUMMARY

Common feedlot problems can be effectively addressed through awareness of options and training of operators and personnel. Operators should recognize options for therapy and continue to refine their skills. It is important to recognize variations in history and signalment and adjust to the situation. Practice and technique adjustment to accommodate varied patient signalment and history as well as facility provisions will address the welfare expectations shared with the public. Ultimately, a safe and quality product can be provided to the consumer.

REFERENCES

1. Booker CW, Abutarbush SM, Schunict OC, et al. Effect of castration timing, technique, and pain management on health and performance of young feedlot bulls in Alberta. Bovine Practitioner 2009;43:1–11.
2. Repenning PE, Ahola JK, Callan RJ, et al. Impact of oral meloxicam administration before and after band castration on feedlot performance and behavioral response in weanling beef bulls. J Anim Sci 2013;91:4965–74.
3. Bretschneider G. Effects of age and method of castration on performance and stress response of beef cattle: a review. Livestock Prod Sci 2005;97:89–100.
4. Rust RL, Thomson DU, Loneragan GH, et al. Effect of different castration methods on growth, performance, and behavior responses of postpubertal beef bulls. Bovine Pract 2009;41:111–18.
5. Pieler D, Peinhopf W, Becher AC, et al. Physiological and behavioral stress parameters in calves in response of partial scrotal resection, orchidectomy and Burdizzo castration. J Dairy Sci 2013;96:6378–89.
6. Dockweiler JC, Coetzee JF, Edwards-Callaway LN, et al. Effect of castration method on neurohormonal and electroencephalographic stress indicators in Holstein calves of different ages. J Dairy Sci 2013;96:4340–54.
7. Moya D, Gonzalez LA, Janzen E, et al. Effects of castration method and frequency of intramuscular injections of ketoprofen on behavioral and physiological indicators of pain in beef cattle. J Anim Sci 2014;92:1686–97.
8. Coetzee JF. A review of pain assessment techniques and pharmacological approaches to pain relief after bovine castration: practical implications for cattle production in the United States. Appl Anim Behav Sci 2011;135:192–213.
9. Lomax S, Windsor PA. Topical anesthesia mitigates the pain of castration in beef calves. J Anim Sci 2013;91:4945–52.
10. Coetzee JF, Gehring R, Tarus-Sanf J, et al. Effect of sub-anesthetic xylazine and ketamine ('ketamine stun') administered to calves immediately prior to castration. Vet Anaesth Analgesia 2010;37:566–78.
11. Anderson DE, Edmondson MA. Prevention and management of surgical pain in cattle. Vet Clin North Am Food Anim Pract 2013;29:157–84. Elsevier Inc.
12. Anderson DE, Muir WW. Pain management in ruminants. Vet Clin North Am 2005; 21:19–31.

13. Coetzee JF. A review of analgesic compounds used in food animals in the United States. Vet Clin North Am Food Anim Pract 2013;29:11–28. Elsevier Inc.
14. Magrath LA, Magrath JM. Tetanus in calves from elastration. J Am Vet Med Assoc 1954;125:451.
15. Skarda RT. Techniques of local analgesia in ruminants and swine. Vet Clin North Am Food Anim Pract 1986;2:621–63.
16. Gonzalez LA, -Schwartzkopf-Genswein KS, Caulkett NA, et al. Pain mitigation after band castration of beef calves and its effects on performance, behaviour, Escherichia coli, and salivary cortisol. J Anim Sci 2010;88:802–10.
17. Currah JM, Hendrick SH, Stookey JM. The behavioral assessment and alleviation of pain associated with castration in beef calves treated with flunixin meglumine and caudal lidocaine epidural anesthesia with epinephrine. Can Vet J 2009;50:375–82.
18. Ting STL, Barley B, Hughes JML, et al. Effect of ketoprofen, lidocaine local anesthesia, and combined xylazine and lidocaine caudal epidural anesthesia during castration of beef cattle on stress responses, immunity, growth, and behavior. J Anim Sci 2003;81:1281–93.
19. Meyer H, Starke A, Kehler W, et al. High caudal epidural anesthesia with local anaesthetics or α2-agonists in calves. J Vet Med A Physiol Pathol Clin Med 2007;54:384–9.
20. Stilwell G, Lima MS, Broom DM. Effects of nonsteroidal anti-inflammatory drugs on long-term pain in calves castrated by use of an external clamping technique following epidural anesthesia. Am J Vet Res 2008;69(6):744–50.
21. Roussel AJ, Navarre CB. Fluid therapy, transfusion, and shock therapy. In: Rings A, editor. Current veterinary therapy – food animal practice. St Louis (MO): Saunders Elsevier; 2009. p. 532–3.
22. Mintline EM, Varga A, Banuelos J, et al. Healing of surgical castration wounds: a description and an evaluation of flunixin. J Anim Sci 2014;92:5659–65.
23. Ballou MA, Sutherland MA, Brooks TA, et al. Administration of anesthetic and analgesic prevent the suppression of many leukocyte responses following surgical castration and physical dehorning. Vet Immunol Immunopathol 2013;151:285–93.
24. Wythes JR, Horder JC, Lapworth JW, et al. Effect of tipped horns on cattle bruising. Vet Rec 1979;104(17):390–2.
25. Neely CD, Thomson DU, Kerr CA, et al. Effects of three dehorning techniques on behavior and wound healing in feedlot cattle. J Anim Sci 2014;92:2225–9.
26. Miesner MD. Bovine surgery of the skin. Vet Clin North Am Food Anim Pract 2008;24:517–26. Elsevier Inc.
27. Nichols S. Tracheotomy and tracheostomy tube placement in cattle. Vet Clin North Am Food Anim Pract 2008;24:307–17. Elsevier Inc.
28. Jensen R, Lauerman LH, Braddy PM, et al. Laryngeal contact ulcers in feedlot cattle. Vet Pathol 1980;17:667–71.
29. Lekeux P, Art T. Functional changes induced by necrotic laryngitis in double muscled calves. Vet Rec 1987;121:353.
30. Plenderleith RWJ. Treatment of cattle, sheep, and horses with lincomycin: case studies. Vet Rec 1988;122:112–3.
31. Fischer W. Experiences with surgical treatment of the larynx in cattle with special consideration of calves. Dtsch Tierarztl Wochenschr 1975;82:137–46.
32. Nichols S, Anderson DE. Subtotal or partial unilateral arytenoidectomy for treatment of arytenoid chondritis in five calves. J Am Vet Med Assoc 2009;235:420–5.

33. Kersjes AW, Nemeth F, Rutgers LJE. The neck: larynx and trachea. In: Kersjes AW, Nemeth F, Rutgers LJE, editors. Atlas of large animal surgery. Utrecht Wetenschappelijke uitgeverji Bunge. London: Williams and Wilkins; 1985. p. 23.

34. Gamboa JC, Angel KL, Shoemaker RS, et al. Laryngeal granuloma in a bull. J Am Vet Med Assoc 1992;201:460–2.

35. Sharma SN, Prasad B, Kohli RN. Some techniques for experimental induction of urine retention in bovines. Indian Vet J 1982;59:972–4.

36. Watts C, Cambell JR. Further studies on the effect of total nephrectomy in the bovine. Res Vet Sci 1971;12:234–5.

37. Ewoldt JM, Jones MJ, Miesner MD. Surgery of obstructive urolithiasis in ruminants. Vet Clin North Am Food Anim Pract 2008;24:455–65. Elsevier Inc.

38. Donawick W. Abdominal surgery. In: Amstutz HE, editor. Bovine medicine and surgery, vol. 2, 2nd edition. Santa Barbara (CA): American Veterinary Publications; 1980. p. 1207–20, 1269.

39. Noordsy JL. Rumenotomy in Cattle. Food animal surgery. 2nd edition. Lenexa (KA): Veterinary Medicine Pub. Co; 1989. p. 105–9. x, 286.

40. Dehghani SN, Ghadrdani AM. Bovine rumenotomy: comparison of four surgical techniques. Can Vet J 1995;36:693–7.

41. Hofmeyr CFB. The digestive system. In: Oehme FW, editor. Textbook of large animal surgery. 2nd edition. Baltimore (MD): Williams & Wilkins; 1988. p. 364–449. xii, 714.

42. Haven ML, Wichtel JJ, Bristol DG, et al. Effects of antibiotic prophylaxis on postoperative complications after rumenotomy in cattle. J Am Vet Med Assoc 1992; 200:1332–5.

43. Buhman MJ, Hungerford LL, Smith DR. An economic risk assessment of the management of pregnant feedlot heifers in the USA. Prev Vet Med 2003;59(4):207–22.

44. Magee AA, Galuppo LD. Comparison of incisional bursting strength of simple continuous and inverted cruciate suture patterns in the equine linea alba. Vet Surg 1999;28(6):442–7.

Surgical Management of Orthopedic and Musculoskeletal Diseases of Feedlot Calves

David E. Anderson, DVM, MS[a],*, Matt D. Miesner, DVM, MS[b]

KEYWORDS

- Pain • Analgesia • Feedlot • Cattle • Lameness • Digit amputation • Pedal osteitis
- Joint ankylosis

KEY POINTS

- Musculoskeletal disorders can be readily recognized and should be addressed early.
- Some disorders are associated with predictable risk factors for development, such as handling methods and facility design, which should be critically evaluated as well.
- The observer should be able to differentiate musculoskeletal disorders of neurologic origin (spastic paresis) from lameness from primary musculoskeletal disease.
- Patient signalment should be part of the decision to treat and/or method of treatment.
- Indicated as well as contraindicated stabilization methods for fractures should be recognized.

PAIN MANAGEMENT

Calves suffering musculoskeletal pain may have acute or chronic pain established. Therefore, the opportunity to perform preemptive pain management eludes the clinician in these cases. However, prevention of pain associated with the surgical procedure is essential to prevent acute exacerbation of a pain condition that might cause the calf to develop a pathologic pain state that is unresponsive to routine drug therapy. Thus, surgical procedures of the foot and limb should be done after induction of local, regional, or general anesthesia. Although general anesthesia can be performed on feedlot calves under field conditions, most procedures are performed with local

The authors have nothing to disclose.
[a] Department of Large Animal Clinical Sciences, College of Veterinary Medicine, University of Tennessee, 2407 River Drive, Knoxville, TN 37996, USA; [b] Department of Clinical Sciences, College of Veterinary Medicine, Kansas State University, A-111 Mosier Hall, Manhattan, KS 66506, USA
* Corresponding author.
E-mail address: dander48@utk.edu

anesthesia administered with 2% lidocaine HCl by local infiltration, epidural infusion, or intravenous regional limb profusion distal to a tourniquet. These techniques are highly effective for obtunding the surgical pain but provide limited postoperative analgesia. The analgesic period of effect for lidocaine is expected to be 60 to 90 minutes. Addition of epinephrine to the lidocaine mixture may extend the clinical period of analgesia. Sedation provides an opportunity to increase analgesia by using complementary drugs such as xylazine (α2 agonist), butorphanol (mixed-agonist/antagonist opioid), and ketamine (neuroleptic, disassociative drug). These drugs, used individually or in various combinations, greatly improve the efficacy of pain management for the surgical procedure but offer little in the way of postoperative pain management.

The most reliable drugs available to feedlot veterinarians for management of musculoskeletal pain are nonsteroidal anti-inflammatory drugs (NSAIDs).[1] These drugs must be used selectively so as not to result in violative residues in meat. In general, recommended meat with holding time for lidocaine and the sedative drugs are less than 5 days. With NSAIDs, meat with holding times range from 24 hours (sodium salicylate) to greater than 60 days (phenylbutazone). Recently, the NSAID meloxicam has become popular as an effective analgesia and anti-inflammatory drug that is inexpensive, can be administered orally, and has a relatively short meat withholding period (< 21 days). However, this drug is not approved for use in food animals and must be prescribed under the regulations stipulated in the animal medical drug use clarification act (AMDUCA)., The dosage most commonly used ranges from 0.5 to 1.0 mg/kg body weight administered every 24 to 72 hours. These NSAID drugs may have benefits to the patient, such as mitigation of pain, lessening of swelling, diminishing inflammation at the incision site and/or damaged tissues, and more rapid recovery after the procedure. Pain, uncontrolled inflammation, excessive swelling, local ischemia, and tissue injury can slow the rate of wound healing, suppress immune system function, and allow the establishment of infection. The use of steroids for management of pain and inflammation associated with surgery is discouraged because of concerns for increased risk of infection at the site of the surgical wound or associated with the disease process necessitating surgery. NSAIDs have been shown to have a beneficial effect on mitigation of pain and maintenance of normal behavioral activities in livestock. The bulk of this research has focused on routine husbandry surgical procedures such as castration and dehorning. In the authors' experience, aspirin (in any form) does not provide sufficient pain mitigation to justify its use with musculoskeletal disease or surgery.[2] The only advantage of sodium salicylate is the rapid elimination and short meat withholding times. This advantage rarely warrants its use because of the negligible clinical effect. Flunixin meglumine is a potent and effective NSAID for use in musculoskeletal disease.[3] However, therapeutic blood concentrations are sustained only for up to 12 hours, and thus, frequent redosing is required. NSAID therapy for treatment of pre-exisitng and severe musculoskeletal disease may require days to weeks of therapy. Thus, NSAIDs that have rapid elimination times are less desirable. Phenylbutazone is effective, has a prolonged elimination time, and can be dosed infrequently, but the drug residue clearance for this drug is prolonged and unpredictable. Therefore, the authors neither use nor advocate using phenylbutazone in feedlot steers. Meloxicam is an increasingly popular NSAID because it possesses desirable potency, slow elimination times, and shorter drug residue clearance intervals even after repeated dosing.[4]

DIGIT AMPUTATION

Toe abscesses and distal limb trauma can result in localized and severe infection within the digit. Deep tissue involvement of the articular surfaces, tendon sheaths, and soft tissue can overwhelm the ability of systemically and locally administered anti-microbial and anti-inflammatory drugs to be of sole benefit. Removal of the digit can be a practical method of treatment. Production life is expected to be shortened with heavier cattle, although postamputation productivity of 10 to 24 months is seen in various production areas.[5,6] Digit removal should not include tissues proximal to the metaphysis of the first phalanx of the affected side, to allow for sufficient weight-bearing stability and limit adverse effects on the metatarsal phalangeal joint. The procedure can be undertaken standing in a squeeze chute or lateral recumbency with proper rope or table restraint.

The affected claw should be clipped and scrubbed for surgical removal. The most effective method of anesthesia is an intravenous regional infusion of 2% lidocaine after tourniquet application to the proximal metatarsus (MT)/metacarpus (MC). Severe inflammation of the soft tissues prevents the action of directly infused lidocaine because of changes in pH and tissue dynamics; therefore, anesthesia must be applied to nerves supplying the area remotely by way of anesthetizing proximal branches of the digital nerves individually or by way of a ring block.

Applying a tourniquet proximal to the proximal MT/MC and infusing lidocaine into a vein distal to the tourniquet allows diffusion of anesthetic to the tissues just distal to the tourniquet. Often, the dorsal common digital vein is infused, as it can be accessed without visualization directly between the digits just proximal to the dorsal interdigital cleft of the claws. About 20 to 25 mL of lidocaine is infused into the vein. A butterfly catheter or short extension on the hypodermic needle improves its ability to remain in the vein during injection during invariable movement by the patient. This method can readily be applied to a standing patient in a squeeze chute with rope restraints. About 3 to 5 minutes are allowed for the anesthetic to take affect before starting amputation.

Methods for removal of the digit can vary. The goal is to remove all the affected tissues distal to the first phalanx (P1) either by disarticulation of the proximal interphalangeal joint or by sharply transecting the distal portion of P1. Ostectomy should be limited to the distal metaphysis of P1, thus retaining the supportive cruciate ligaments shared between the phalanges for stability and limiting stress on the fetlock joint.[7,8] Disarticulation of the proximal interphalangeal joint can be performed, but at least one review showed a decrease in vascular recruitment for wound healing and possibly slower healing time.[9] Before the distal P1 can be removed or proximal interphalangeal joint disarticulated, the soft tissues must be sharply incised with a scalpel blade. The incision first encircles the circumference of the coronary band. In addition to the circumferential incision, 2 perpendicular incisions can be extended proximally, parallel to the dorsal and plantar/palmar pastern or 1 incision extended proximally, abaxial to the pastern. These incisions and soft-tissue reflection allow for visual access to the proximal interphalangeal joint for disarticulation or visualization of the distal P1 for ostectomy while maintaining some soft-tissue coverage of exposed bone after amputation. If all of the affected tissue is removed with the amputation, closure of the remaining skin can be performed. The wound should remain open for drainage otherwise.

Ostectomy of P1 can be performed with obstetric wire or bone saw. A sterilized carpenter's coping saw is effective and easily controllable for ostectomy. Gigli wire placement in the axial interdigital space for ostectomy is practical for standing removal in a squeeze chute. The wire or saw is placed in the axial portion of the coronary incision as close to the bone as possible and angled proximal and abaxial to remove the affected digit distal to P1. Disarticulation of the joint begins abaxial and is continued through the joint with a scalpel. Once the claw is removed, the severed interdigital artery should be identified if possible for ligation, but it may not be seen. If the affected tissue was removed and skin tissue sufficient for closure remains, the skin is closed in a series of cruciate sutures such that the incision can be partially or completely opened should drainage be needed later (**Fig. 1**). If severe cellulitis is present at the time of surgery, skin closure should not be attempted. The area should be bandaged tightly with a compression bandage to provide protection and promote hemostasis. The bandage can be removed and or changed every 3 to 5 days until granulation is present. The wound should be left open once sufficient granulation and protection has occurred (**Fig. 2**).

ANKYLOSIS OF THE DISTAL INTERPHALANGEAL JOINT

The techniques for ankylosis of the distal interphalangeal (DIP) joint differ by their surgical approach. The choice of a technique should be based on the anatomic structure infected and the location of existing draining tracts. Intact ligaments and tendons should be preserved, when possible, to keep the affected digit stable during the ankylosis procedure.

Ankylosis of the DIP joint has been described extensively in the literature.[10–13] For unknown reasons, those techniques have been used sparingly in North America.[14,15] The advantages of ankylosis of the DIP joint compared with digit amputation are that cattle have a longer production life, the outcome is superior for heavy animals, return to production is better when the hind lateral or front medial digit are affected, and the healing result is more cosmetic and mechanically stable. Disadvantages are that it is more expensive and technically demanding, more postoperative care is needed, and cattle return slower to previous production because of the pain engendered by the procedure and the long process of ankylosis. The techniques described in the German literature are used mostly in cattle with septic arthritis of the DIP secondary to ascending infection from a complicated sole ulcer at the junction of the sole and heel.[10–13] The distal sesamoid bone and its synovial bursa and the tendinous portion of deep digital flexor (DDF) muscle and its tendon sheath usually are infected and necrotic when the origin of the septic DIP joint is a complicated sole ulcer.

Plantar (Heel Bulb) Approach to Ankylosis

The surgery is performed under sedation and intravenous regional anesthesia. Cattle are restrained in a foot trimming chute or in lateral recumbency with the affected leg

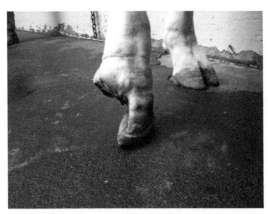

Fig. 1. Lateral claw amputation due to a septic P3 (coffin) joint infection only and wound sutured.

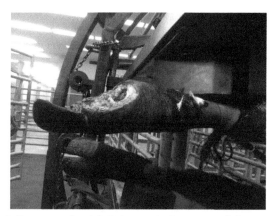

Fig. 2. Claw amputation approximately 5 days post–claw removal. A second bandage will be applied for another 3 to 5 days. Eventually wound to be left open to heal after granulation covers wound completely. Note distal portion of the first phalanx is still exposed in the center of the granulating bed.

uppermost. The plantar or palmar portion of the sole and the heel should be pared away until the sole can be indented easily. In severe and extensive infection of the DIP joint originating from solar lesions, the distal sesamoid bone and the joint can be felt through the wound, and the sole can be indented easily. The distal limb is prepared aseptically. A vertical incision starting 2 cm distal to the accessory digit is made along the axis of the plantar or palmar aspect of the proximal phalanx and continued in an elliptical fashion around the necrotic area of the heel and sole junction. The tendinous portion of the DDF muscle is cut from its insertion on the distal phalanx and resected proximally at about 2 to 3 in (5–7.6 cm) from its insertion. The distal sesamoid bone is then exposed. If necrotic, it is removed easily with a rongeur. If not, the 2 collateral ligaments and the distal ligaments are resected with a scalpel blade. The DIP joint then is exposed. Debridement of the joint from the solar wound and through the dorsal hoof wall, 1 cm distal to the coronary band, is performed with a 1.3-cm-diameter drill bit. The joint is curetted, and copious lavage is done with isotonic solution.

If the tendon sheath or the tendinous portion of the superficial digital flexor (SDF) muscle is infected, the incision is extended 2 to 3 cm proximal to the accessory digit, allowing debridement and drainage. A wooden block is apposed with polymethylmethacrylate acrylic (PMMA) on the healthy digit of the affected limb, and the claws are wired together with the affected digit in slight flexion. The wound is bandaged, and wound lavage is done every other day, if possible. Systemic antibiotics are given for 2 to 3 weeks and NSAIDs administered as needed for the first 2 weeks.

Köstlin and Nuss[12] have reported a success rate of 85.8% on 281 cattle with this technique. More than 50% returned to their previous level of production. In 39 of 281 cattle, the treatment failed because of uncontrolled infection or other unrelated diseases. Thirty-nine percent of the cattle showed slight hoof abnormalities (hyperextension of the digit) secondary to the loss of the tendinous portion of the DDF muscle. This technique provides good visualization of the DIP joint, excellent drainage, and a good long-term prognosis. However, the approach to the joint is difficult. Even if not affected by the septic process, the tendinous portion of the DDF muscle and the distal sesamoid bone have to be resected, as well as the tendon sheath, creating an unnecessary instability of the joint.

A variation of this technique has been reported by Greenough and Ferguson.[15] The approach consists of a horizontal incision around the circumference of the heel 1 cm distal to the skin-horn junction. A wedge of hypodermic tissue and tendon is resected, providing visualization of the navicular bone. The navicular bone is resected, as described earlier, and the digit is extended to provide a good view of the DIP joint. After debridement and lavage of the joint, the incision can be sutured and bandaged. A wooden block is applied with PMMA on the healthy digit of the affected limb. This technique provides better visualization of the DIP joint and, ideally, does not invade the tendon sheath when it is not necessary.

Ankylosis of the Distal Interphalangeal Joint Through the Hoof Wall (Abaxial Approach)

In this technique, an orthopedic drill with a 6- to 12-mm drill bit is used to create a tunnel through the abaxial hoof wall at the level of the DIP joint. The drill is passed through the DIP joint and exited through the dorsoaxial interdigital space distal to the coronary band.[16] The entry site for the drill bit is estimated as the intersection of 2 imaginary lines, one drawn parallel to the coronary band approximately one-third the distance from the coronary band to the sole and the other line drawn perpendicular to the coronary band approximately half the distance from the heel bulb to the dorsal hoof wall. This approach is easy to perform, but the exit site of the drill bit is difficult to control, especially if the animal is not well restrained. Debridement of the cartilage and necrotic bone also is difficult to assess. The defect in the hoof wall remains open to facilitate drainage; thus, the hoof wall is weakened by this technique. The authors have not observed specific hoof wall complications of this technique, but cattle should be confined to a small area with excellent footing during the early stages of healing.

Steiner and Zulauf[17] proposed an alternative to this method. They performed a precise abaxial hoof wall excision using a fine rotating burr. A hoof wall segment measuring approximately 15 × 40 mm was removed, and the proximal margin of the defect was approximately 1 cm distal to the coronary band. This technique provides a large, rectangular hoof wall defect through which to access the DIP joint. Although access to the joint is superior to the previously described technique, the defect size is substantial.

PEDAL OSTEITIS

Pedal osteitis is defined as a septic process of the distal phalanx. The infection originates from solar trauma (eg, puncture wound, severe abrasion at the toe) or extension of an existing infection around the distal phalanx (eg, DIP joint sepsis, sole ulcer, sole abscess). Pedal osteitis occurs sporadically in a herd. The incidence is expected to be higher in cattle on concrete flooring. Cattle recently placed in a feedlot or without adequate bunker space fight to compete at the feed bunk and their hind digits become abraded on the concrete floor, causing severe abrasion at the toe region and secondary infection.

The sole and infected corium are debrided first. The infected part of the distal phalanx is curetted (**Fig. 3**). Necrotic bone feels more brittle than normal bone. Frequent probing of the lesion is important to avoid communication with the DIP joint. Lavage is performed, and the wound is bandaged. A wooden block is applied on the healthy digit of the affected limb. Bandaging and lavage should be continued until the infection is controlled and granulation tissue covers the distal phalanx. Prognosis is good if the infection is limited to the distal phalanx. Amputation could be performed for economic reasons or if the infection is too extensive.

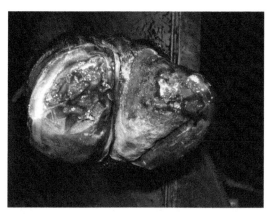

Fig. 3. Angus heifer's foot after resection of the cranial aspect of the sole, dorsal hoof wall, and distal one-fourth of the pedal bone (P3). The heifer suffered toxic laminitis followed by sepsis resulting in pedal osteitis.

FRACTURE MANAGEMENT

The location of the fracture, presence of soft tissue and neurovascular trauma, closed or open fracture environment, behavioral nature of the animal, and experience of the veterinarian are important factors for considering what type of treatment is chosen.[18] Physical examination should be conducted and the patient made safe from continued trauma. Young calves may suffer life-threatening hemorrhage after femur fracture if the femoral artery has been lacerated. Temporary stabilization of limb fractures may be performed before moving the animal or attempting to get the animal to stand. As a general rule, fractures below the level of the midradius or midtibia may be temporarily stabilized with splints or casts. Stabilization of fractures proximal to this level are more likely to become exacerbated by soft-tissue trauma, damage to neurovascular structures, or compounding of the fracture as a result of the coaptation and therefore may not be advisable. In the authors' experience, proximal limb fractures such as those involving the humerus or femur, are best managed without application of any bandage or appliance to the limb. The affected animal is placed in a quiet area, sedated if needed, and allowed to lay down on their own. Cattle may self-protect these proximal limb fractures by remaining quiet and recumbent until a treatment plan can be devised.

Splinting

External coaptation for temporary stabilization of the fracture may be done by using 2 splints or a cast. Two boards or pieces of a large polyvinyl chloride pipe cut in half and placed 90° to each other (eg, caudal and lateral aspect of the limb) create a stable external coaptation. A padded bandage is placed on the limb, the splints are positioned, and an elastic tape is applied firmly. Circular clamps (eg, hose clamps) may be used to achieve firm placement of the splints on the limb. The injury should be centered within the coaptation with as much support proximal and distal to the injury as possible. All external coaptation devices should extend to the ground. For injuries distal to the carpus or hock, the splints should be placed to the level of the proximal radius or tibia, respectively. For injuries proximal to the carpus or hock and distal to the midradius or midtibia, the lateral splint should extend to the level of the proximal scapula or pelvis, respectively.

Casting

Half-limb casts (short casts) can be used for immobilization of fractures of the distal MC or MT. The cast is placed from a point immediately distal to the carpus or hock and extending to the ground and encasing the foot. Encasing the foot helps to ensure that ground reaction forces do not cause displacement of the fracture within the cast. Before placement of the fiberglass cast, a double layer of stockinette is rolled onto the limb and padding is applied in a ring around where the top of the cast ends, over any bony prominences, and between the dew claws and the pastern. The remainder of the limb is not padded in most cases because thick padding compresses within the cast and results in space for the limb to move within the cast, which may result in displacement of the fracture. Full-limb casts are used for fractures occurring at or proximal to the mid-MC or MT but distal to the midradius or midtibia. Full-limb casts are placed in a manner similar to half-limb casts, but the bony prominences of the accessory carpal bone, styloid process of the ulna, calcaneous, and medial and lateral maleolus of the tibia must be padded.

Placement of the cast is facilitated by use of rope restraint, sedation, or anesthesia as needed. An assistant should help to maintain alignment of the limb during application, being sure to check the position of the limb in cranial to caudal (sagittal) and lateral to medial (frontal) planes. Tension on the limb during casting may be achieved by placing wires through holes drilled in the hoof wall and applying tension. The holes should be placed such that the hoof is positioned in a slightly flexed position.

The thickness of the cast is usually based on clinical judgment. Casts 6 to 8 layers thick may be adequate for calves less than 150 kg body weight, 10 to 12 layers for calves 150 to 300 kg, and 12 to 14 layers for calves 300 to 600 kg. Casts used on the hind limbs must be made thicker because of stress concentration by the angulation of the hock. Incorporation of metal rods within the cast (2 rods placed 90° to each other) can increase the strength of the cast but is needed only in the largest of patients. Newer fiberglass casting materials are more resistant to breaking and do not weaken when wet if sufficient cast material is used compared with plaster of paris casting materials. Use of a walking bar (U-shaped bar placed under the hoof and incorporated into the cast) increases distribution of loading forces into the cast and away from the distal limb, but the foot should always be included in the cast.

Casts may be maintained in calves for 4 to 6 weeks without being changed. Physeal fractures are usually healed within 4 weeks, but nonphyseal fractures often require 6 weeks to heal.

Thomas Splint and Cast Combination

Use of a Thomas splint and cast combination is appropriate for fractures proximal to the midradius and midtibia but distal to the elbow or stifle.[19] The length of the splint should be measured while the animal is standing and by using the normal limb for measurements. An appropriate splint is chosen or constructed, and the patient is placed into lateral recumbency (rope restraint, sedation, and/or anesthesia). The fracture is reduced and a cast applied from the distal MC or MT to the level of the proximal radius or tibia. The splint is placed on the limb, the foot is attached to the base of the splint by drilling holes in the hoof walls and wiring the foot to the splint base, and casting tape is used to attach the cast to the splint frame. The limb cast should be firmly attached to the splint frame to prevent rotation of the limb along the splint during ambulation. The hoop of the splint must be firmly placed into the axilla or groin to allow maximal weight transference, and, therefore, the hoop must be heavily padded (**Fig. 4**). Cattle having a Thomas splint-cast should be assisted to stand for 3 to

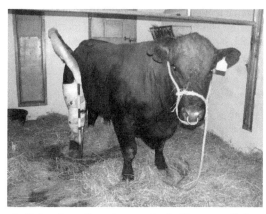

Fig. 4. Adult Angus bull standing after placement of a Thomas splint-cast for management of a proximal tibia fracture.

5 days until they learn how to rise under their own power. These patients must be checked several times daily to ensure that they have not laid down on top of the splint. Often, patients are not able to rise after lying down on the splint, and life-threatening rumen tympany may occur if they remain trapped for a prolonged period.

Transfixation Pinning and Casting and External Skeletal Fixation

Transfixation pinning and casting may be applied either as a hanging limb pin cast or as an external skeletal fixator.[18] Hanging limb pin cast refers to placement of transfixing, or transcortical, pins through the bone proximal to the injury, followed by application of a full-limb cast. The body weight is transferred into the cast by the pins and transmitted through the cast to the ground. Therefore, the distal limb hangs inside of the pin-cast. Pin-casts also may be used for external skeletal fixation (ESF) by placing transfixation pins proximal and distal to the injury.

Pin selection is made based on the body weight of the animal, the size of the bone involved, and the configuration of the fracture. In general, 3/32- to 1/8-in (2.4–3.2 mm) pins are used in calves weighing less than 100 kg, 1/8- to 3/16-in (3.2–4.8 mm) pins are used in cattle weighing 100 to 300 kg, 3/16- to 1/4-inch (4.8 to 6.4 mm) pins are used in cattle weighing 300 to 600 kg, and 1/4-inch (6.4 mm) pins are used in cattle weighing more than 600 kg. Pins should be placed in the bone such that they are separated by a minimum of 6 times the diameter of the pin (eg, two 4.8-mm diameter pins should be placed a minimum of 30 mm apart). This distance minimizes the risk of the concentration of mechanical forces between the 2 pins (stress riser effect). Before pin insertion, a hole should be predrilled through the bone to accommodate the pin. This hole should not be smaller than 0.5 mm of the diameter of the pin (eg, 2.7-mm predrilled hole for a 3.2-mm pin). Veterinary orthopedic pins, in general, are not designed to drill while being inserted. Therefore, significant thermal and mechanical injury occurs in the bone during insertion. Predrilling, using an orthopedic drill bit, prevents or limits this injury.

Closed Versus Open Fractures

Overall, closed fractures without damage to the blood supply to the limb have a good to excellent prognosis for healing in cattle. The prognosis for success is less for older cattle or cattle of high body weight. Open fractures have a guarded prognosis for healing in cattle. The success rate depends on the severity of soft-tissue damage, the bone affected, the age of the patient, the duration and degree of contamination of the wound, and the economic limitations placed on fracture management. Prolonged antibiotic therapy is indicated, and open wound management is preferable to enclosing the wound within a cast. Young calves with open fractures are prone to nonunion or delayed union. Prolonged antibiotic therapy for open fractures increases the risk of meat adulteration, violative residues, and poor-quality carcass yields.

Metacarpus and Metatarsus III/IV

Fractures involving the MC or MT III/IV are the most common fractures to occur in food animals. Closed fracture of the distal physis of the MC or MT may be treated using a half-limb cast. Closed fracture of the middle portion of the MC or MT may be treated with a full-limb cast. Open fractures in mature cattle may be treated by thoroughly debriding, cleaning, and flushing the wound; applying a full-limb cast; and administering antibiotics for 10 to 14 days. Bone sequestra are often associated with open fractures of the MC and MT. Bone healing may not occur until sequestra have been removed.

Humerus

Nonarticular, minimally displaced fractures of the humerus are best treated by stall confinement. The prognosis for healing the fracture with stall confinement is good (>50%) in calves less than 500 kg.

Radius and Ulna

Closed fractures of the distal physis of the radius may be treated by a full-limb cast and has a good prognosis for success. Fracture of the midradius and ulna requires use of a Thomas splint-cast, transfixation pin-cast, or bone plate. The prognosis for healing is good, but significant contralateral limb injury may occur in animals treated by Thomas splint-cast. Transfixation pinning and casting has a good to excellent prognosis, with minimal risk of permanent injury to the contralateral limb. Where applicable and economical, the author prefers to treat fractures of the radius and ulna using transfixation pinning and casting.

Tibia

Tibia fractures are usually caused by trauma. Fracture of the distal physis of the tibia may be treated with a full-limb cast, but these fractures are uncommon. Fracture of the middle portion of the tibia occurs most often and may be treated by Thomas splint-cast or transfixation pinning and casting. Thomas splint-casts have a good prognosis for bone healing but have a high rate of injury to the contralateral limb.[19] Transfixation pin-casts have a good to excellent prognosis for healing and minimal problems with contralateral limb injury.

Complications of Fracture Management

The most common complications of fracture injury are sepsis, nerve injury, and vascular injury. The most common complications of fracture treatment are cast or splint sores, breakdown injury in the contralateral limb, and malunion. Septic nonunion may occur from a combination of factors involved with fracture injury and fracture treatment. Nerve and vascular injury can be minimized by appropriate fracture immobilization before transporting the animal for achieving definitive fracture treatment. Sepsis can be minimized by close attention to detail, thorough cleaning of the fracture site, and selection of appropriate antimicrobial drugs. Malunion can be prevented by effective closed reduction and stabilization. Contralateral limb injury can be prevented by strict confinement of the animal during convalescence, frequent monitoring, removal of external coaptation at the earliest appropriate time, and client education for fracture patient management. When possible, environmental management should be used to limit risk factors for feedlot fractures (eg, slippery flooring, obstacles in working area, aggressive handling, overcrowding, mixing of heifers/bulls/steers).

TENDON DISORDERS

Tendon disorders are a recognized cause of locomotor dysfunction in cattle, but the prevalence of lameness caused by tendon injury presently is unknown. One study indicated tendon involvement in 21% of limb lesions.[20] Another study reported that muscle and/or tendon lesions accounted for 74% of upper limb injuries in the forelimb and 7.8% in the hind limb.[21] Tendon injuries causing loss of a production animal or a decreased level of production result in significant economic loss.

Spastic Paresis

Spastic paresis is a progressive neuromuscular disease that occurs in dairy, beef, and crossbred cattle. Signs of spastic paresis usually appear at a few weeks to several months of age.[22] Spastic contractions of one or both gastrocnemius muscles and SDF tendons lead to hyperextension of the hock. The affected leg is extended caudally and is advanced in a swinging motion. With progression of the disease, the foot often may not touch the ground, and gluteal muscle atrophy occurs. Palpation of the limb shows that the gastrocnemius muscle is hard and rigid, but flexion of the hock is not painful. The base of the tail often is elevated. Initially, few if any systemic effects result from the condition. With its progression, however, the animal may remain recumbent for a longer period and loses weight. Outcomes after treatment of spastic paresis is highly variable, and calves often must be slaughtered prematurely.

Two techniques have been described: tibial neurectomy or transection of a portion of the gastrocnemius and superficial flexor tendons.[23,24] Partial or complete tibial neurectomy is aesthetically more pleasing. The procedure can be performed under sedation and epidural anesthesia or under general anesthesia with the animal placed in lateral recumbency with the affected leg uppermost. The tibial nerve is found via a lateral incision through the biceps femoris muscle. The tibial nerve is located caudal to the peroneal nerve. The tibial nerve is isolated, and its different branches are stimulated electrically to evaluate the corresponding muscle contraction. A 3-cm-long segment is excised from each of the 2 nerve branches to the gastrocnemius. Closure is routine. Only 1 leg should be operated on at a time to assess the efficacy of the procedure. Partial tibial neurectomy has resulted in good to excellent results in 131 of 138 (95%) calves.[23] The authors have performed complete and partial tibial neurectomy on a large number of calves effected with spastic paresis. Although clinical improvement is obvious, the results are suboptimal, are temporary usually lasting 4 to 6 months, and often do not allow the calf to return to a level of productive performance intended by the owner.

Transection of a portion of the gastrocnemius and SDF tendons is performed after sedation, with the animal placed in lateral recumbency and with the affected leg uppermost.[24] The leg is surgically prepared from the mid-MT to the stifle, and 2% lidocaine is locally infiltrated over a 10-cm length proximal to the calcaneus and over the cranial border of the lateral aspect of the calcaneal tendon. The 2 tendons of insertion of the gastrocnemius muscle (lateral and medial head of the gastrocnemius muscle) and half of the SDF tendons are transected for a length of 2 cm, approximately 6 cm proximal to the point of the hock. The subcutis is closed with a simple continuous pattern, followed by a layer of simple uninterrupted skin sutures of nonabsorbable monofilament material. A bandage is applied over the surgical site for 5 days, and the skin sutures are removed after 14 days.

The immediate effect of surgery is that the hock becomes profoundly flexed and the MT becomes nearly parallel to the ground. Fibrous unions generally develop between the tendon ends, and limb posture returns in 4 to 6 weeks. Spasticity often returns slowly over several months. The authors have performed complete or partial gastrocnemius tenotomy on a large number of calves. Although clinical improvement is obvious, the results are temporary, usually lasting 4 to 6 months and often do not allow the calf to return to a level of productive performance expected by the owner. This procedure can easily be done in field conditions and may be preferred as compared with tibial neurectomy because of the lower expense associated with the procedure.

Tendon Laceration

Tendon laceration is an uncommon cause of lameness in cattle and occurs most commonly when the calf falls onto or kicks a sharp object. The rear limbs are affected most commonly.[25] Typically an open wound with contamination or infection is present at the site of tendon rupture. Feedlot cattle that are housed in concentrated environments with frequent exposure to farm machinery may have greater prevalence of tendon injuries. Lacerations occur most commonly in a single hind limb at the level of the mid-MT. Spontaneous tendon rupture is most commonly associated with breeding accidents, bull fights, or peer trauma and usually involves the gastrocnemius muscle-tendon unit. Spontaneous rupture of the gastrocnemius muscle usually occurs at the junction of the muscle fibers and tendon.[25–29] Rupture of the gastrocnemius tendon adjacent to the insertion on the tuber calcaneus may be caused by direct trauma.

Treatment of Tendon Disruption

Flexor tendon lacerations can be managed successfully in cattle by external coaptation, alone. Economic costs associated with treatment and prolonged convalescence should be discussed with the owner before attempting therapy. The owner's expectation for long-term productivity should include the likelihood of persistent lameness.

Options for treatment of tendon laceration in feedlot cattle include stall rest, use of a wooden or rubber block on the healthy digit, and cast application. The location of the lesion, individual tendon involvement, and concurrent injuries are important factors for treatment selection.[30] Stall confinement may be adequate for incomplete lacerations and partial disruption of the gastrocnemius muscle or tendon. Application of a wooden block is useful when disruption of the branches of the DDF tendons (III or IV) to a single digit are affected. A full-limb or half-limb cast may be indicated for injuries disrupting the flexor tendons to both digits of the same limb. Stall rest, use of a wooden block, and external coaptation of the limb result in healing of the tendon by scar tissue formation.

Flexor tendon laceration located distal to the hock may be treated with application of a cast including the foot and extending to the level of the hock but not spanning the hock.[31,32] The fetlock may be flexed during casting to release tension from the tendons and allow closer apposition of the tendon ends. Alternatively, the limb may be cast in a normal, standing position. The authors recommend that the cast be maintained for 3 to 4 weeks longer than when a flexed fetlock cast is used. The fetlock must be lightly padded on the dorsal and palmar/plantar aspect to protect the limb from pressure-induced cast sores (ulcerations).

Laceration of the calcaneal tendon often requires suture reconstruction of the tendon (tenorrhaphy) in addition to application of a cast including the foot and extending to the proximal tibia (level of the tibial crest). Suture repair (tenorrhaphy) of transected tendons in addition to external coaptation achieves a more mature scar and a stronger scar-tendon unit more rapidly than does healing by second intention. Nylon, polydioxanon, and polyglyconate are the most common suture material used for tendon repair. The portion of the cast spanning the hock must be thicker than the remainder of the cast to prevent breakage of the cast at this point. Reinforcing splints may provide a stronger construct and if used should be placed on the tension and compression sides of the limb. Thomas splints may be used to stabilize gastrocnemius muscle-tendon disruption, but in the authors' experience, the results have been poor. A full-limb cast is preferred when the disruption is close to the calcaneus. The authors recommend that external coaptation be maintained for a minimum of 45 days after complete transection of flexor tendons. After cast removal, a block may be used to elevate the heel and stall confinement should be continued for 2 to 4 weeks after cast removal. The prognosis for tendon rupture in cattle is considered good for injuries involving the SDF tendon alone. In the authors' experience, the prognosis for survival and for long-term productivity of cattle with traumatic rupture of the digital flexor tendons (SDF and/or DDF and/or suspensory ligament [SL]) is fair to good. Treatment of gastrocnemius tendon rupture has been recommended only for young, lightweight cattle. With complete disruption of the calcaneal tendon or gastrocnemius muscle, prognosis is grave for cattle weighing more than 500 kg and poor for cattle weighing less than 500 kg.

SUMMARY

Musculoskeletal diseases can be addressed in feedlot practice promptly and effectively through awareness and training of disease presentation. Knowledge of basic principles and techniques can effectively eliminate painful or infected sites and stabilize injuries. The operator should also recognize contraindicated applications. Decisions to treat or stall rest should have objective criteria in place to evaluate patient response and recognize ineffective treatment and humane status of the situation.

REFERENCES

1. Coetzee JF. A review of analgesic compounds used in food animals in the United States. Vet Clin North Am Food Anim Pract 2013;29:11–28.
2. Kotchwar JL, Coetzee JF, Anderson DE, et al. Analgesic efficacy of sodium salicylate in an amphotericin B-induced bovine synovitis-arthritis model. J Dairy Sci 2009;92(8):3731–43.
3. Schulz KL, Anderson DE, Coetzee JF, et al. Effect of flunixin meglumine on the amelioration of lameness in dairy steers with amphotericin B-induced transient synovitis-arthritis. Am J Vet Res 2011;72(11):1431–8.
4. Offinger J, Herdtweck S, Rizk A, et al. Postoperative analgesic efficacy of meloxicam in lame dairy cows undergoing resection of the distal interphalangeal joint. J Dairy Sci 2013;96(2):866–76.
5. Pejsa TG, St-Jean G, Hoffsis GF, et al. Digit amputation in cattle: 85 cases (1971-1990). J Am Vet Med Assoc 1993;202:981–4.
6. Funk K. Late results of digit amputation in cattle. Berl Munch Tierarztl Wochenschr 1977;90:152.
7. Turner AS, McIlawraith CW. Techniques in large animal surgery. 2nd edition. Philadelphia: Lea and Febiger; 1989. p. 333.
8. Desrochers A, Anderson DE, St Jean G. Surgical diseases and techniques of the digit. Vet Clin North Am Food Anim Pract 2008;24:535–50.

9. Gogoi SN, Singh AP, Nigam JM. Clinical, radiographic, and angiographic studies following amputation of the digit in bovine. Haryana Agric Univ J Res 1983;3(1): 19–26.

10. Breuer D. A new operative procedure for sole ulcer in cattle. Tierärztl Umsch 1963;18:646.

11. Clemente CH. Contribution to the development of tendon resection and pedal joint resection in cattle. Tierärztl Umsch 1965;20:108.

12. Köstlin RG, Nuss K. Treatment of septic pedal arthritis in cattle by joint resection: results. Tierärztl Prax 1988;16:123.

13. Nuss K, Weaver MP. Resection of the distal interphalangeal joint in cattle: an alternative to digit amputation. Vet Rec 1991;128:540.

14. Blislager AT, Baines SJ, Bowman KF. Excision of the distal sesamoid bone for treatment of infection of the digit in a heifer. J Am Vet Med Assoc 1905;201:1992.

15. Greenough PR, Ferguson JG. Alternatives to amputation. Vet Clin North Am Food Anim Pract 1985;1(1):195–203. In: Ferguson JG, editor. Philadelphia: WB Saunders.

16. Greenough PR, MacCallum FJ, Weaver AD. Lameness in cattle. 2nd edition. Philadelphia: Lippincott; 1981.

17. Steiner A, Zulauf M. Fenestration of the abaxial hoof wall and implantation of gentamicin-impregnated collagen sponges for treatment of septic arthritis of the distal interphalangeal joint in cattle. Vet Rec 2001;149:516–8.

18. Anderson DE, St-Jean G. External skeletal fixation in ruminants. Vet Clin North Am Food Anim Pract 1996;12:117–52.

19. Anderson DE, St-Jean G, Vestweber JG, et al. Use of a Thomas splint-cast combination for stabilization of tibial fractures in cattle: 21 cases (1973-1993). Agri-Pract 1994;15:16–23.

20. Russell AM, Rowlands GJ, Shaw SR, et al. Survey of lameness in British dairy cattle. Vet Rec 1982;111:155–60.

21. Arkins S. Lameness in dairy cows. Ir Vet J 1981;35:135–40.

22. Leipold HW, Huston K, Guffy MM, et al. Spastic paresis in beef shorthorn cattle. J Am Vet Med Assoc 1967;151:598–601.

23. Vlaminck L, De Moor A, Martens A, et al. Partial tibial neurectomy in 113 Belgian blue calves with spastic paresis. Vet Rec 2000;147(1):16–9.

24. Weaver AD, St-Jean G, Steiner A. Spastic paresis. In: Weaver AD, St-Jean G, Steiner A, editors. Bovine Surgery and Lameness (2nd edition). Ames (IA): Blackwell Publishing; 2005. p. 246–8.

25. Greenough PR, Maccallum FJ, Weaver AD. Diseases of muscles. In: Greenough PR, Maccallum FJ, Weaver AD, editors. Lameness in cattle. Philadelphia: Lippincott; 1981. p. 363–73.

26. Homey FD, Amstutz HE. Musculoskeletal system. In: Amstutz HE, editor. Bovine medicine and surgery, vol. 2. Santa Barbara (CA): American Veterinary Publications; 1980. p. 863–85.

27. Johnson JH. The musculoskeletal system (muscles and tendons). In: Oehme FW, editor. Textbook of large animal surgery. 2nd edition. Baltimore (MD): Williams & Wilkins; 1988. p. 231–61.

28. Turner AS. Large animal orthopedics. In: Jennings PB, editor. The practice of large animal surgery, vol. 2. Philadelphia: Saunders; 1984. p. 768–949.

29. Wheat JD, Asbury AC. Rupture of the gastrocnemius muscle in a cow – a case report. J Am Vet Med Assoc 1958;132:331–2.

30. Stashak TA. Lameness. In: Stashak TS, editor. Adam's lameness in horses. 4th edition. Philadelphia: Lea and Febiger; 1987. p. 764–7.

31. Wilson DC, Vanderby R. An evaluation of six synthetic casting materials: strength 01 cylinders in bending. Vet Surg 1995;24:55–9.
32. Wilson DC, Vanderby R. An evaluation of fiberglass application techniques. Vet Surg 1995;24:118–21.

Treatment of Calves with Bovine Respiratory Disease
Duration of Therapy and Posttreatment Intervals

Michael D. Apley, DVM, PhD

KEYWORDS

- Bovine • Respiratory disease • Therapy • Duration • Posttreatment interval

KEY POINTS

- Data are lacking to define the optimal duration of antimicrobial exposure for bovine respiratory disease (BRD).
- Human pneumonia studies evaluating optimal antimicrobial duration have consistently been unable to demonstrate differences between shorter and longer durations evaluated in the studies.
- Defining the duration of antimicrobial effect, and therefore when success/failure definitions should be applied, based on pharmacokinetics and pharmacodynamics may mislead us as to the optimal posttreatment interval (PTI).
- PTI studies for BRD suggest 7 days may be a default PTI unless data to indicate otherwise are available.
- The industry needs additional PTI studies to provide sufficient periods of drug exposure to optimize clinical success while still attempting to control exposure and minimizing selection for resistant pathogens.

INTRODUCTION

The 3 most basic components of treating any disease are the criteria for making the decision to treat, the treatment regimen, and then the criteria for determining the success or failure. The advent of single injection antimicrobials for bovine respiratory disease (BRD) has brought about an emphasis on the interval between therapy administration and applying success and failure criteria, initially based on an estimate of when therapeutic effects waned, and later confirmed by randomized clinical trials. This period between therapeutic application and evaluation of success or failure is known as the posttreatment interval (PTI). Before these single-injection antimicrobials,

The author has nothing to disclose.
Department of Clinical Sciences, Kansas State University College of Veterinary Medicine, 1800 Denison Avenue, Manhattan, KS 66506, USA
E-mail address: mapley@vet.ksu.edu

Vet Clin Food Anim 31 (2015) 441–453
http://dx.doi.org/10.1016/j.cvfa.2015.06.001
0749-0720/15/$ – see front matter © 2015 Elsevier Inc. All rights reserved.

the PTI for BRD antimicrobials administered on a daily basis was typically the next day after cessation of therapy. Were we right?

This article looks at available evidence that may inform us as to how long antimicrobial exposure should persist, examines how we have classically determined the "duration of therapy" for antimicrobials in the treatment of BRD, and summarizes available data that may drive decisions on the optimal duration of the PTI.

DURATION OF THERAPY: HOW LONG SHOULD IT BE?

The available data from both human and veterinary medicine pertaining to optimal duration of respiratory disease therapy are quite limited. In fact, the data are limited for any disease in any species. Recent emphasis on duration of therapy in human medicine has been driven by the need to balance therapeutic efficacy with minimizing exposure in an attempt to slow the development of antimicrobial resistance in both the target pathogen and the microbiota of the patient. Recent reports of antimicrobial resistance in diagnostic laboratory isolates from BRD suggest that a similar approach may be well-advised for at least some cattle production system flows.[1]

Looking for parallels in human medicine may inform our thinking and investigations in veterinary medicine. The lack of clear guidance for duration of therapy in human respiratory disease mirrors that of BRD. Recent reviews have pointed out the limited data available for duration of therapy for respiratory disease in humans.[2,3] A Cochrane Database Systematic Review of human randomized clinical trials concluded that a 7- to 8-day course of antibiotic therapy is more appropriate than 10 to 15 days in patients with ventilator-associated pneumonia not associated with a nonfermenting Gram negative bacteria.[4] When nonfermenting Gram negative bacteria were present in ventilator-associated pneumonia, the clinical trials suggested that increased recurrence of disease occurred after short-term therapy, although all other measured parameters were equal. This review illustrates that many factors contribute to the decision of duration of therapy, including type of pneumonia, patient condition, pathogen, and drug regimen.

A summary of individual clinical trials conducted in relation to human respiratory disease therapy is provided in **Table 1**. Although it is important to note that these studies consist of a different mammalian species with different pulmonary characteristics and different pathogens, there is also a pattern in the results which is of great interest. Five of these human studies were conducted with different durations of the same regimen. In the first study, oral amoxicillin was evaluated for 5 days after a 3-day intravenous course as compared with a placebo oral follow-up regimen by el Moussaoui and colleagues.[5] File and colleagues[6] evaluated gemifolxacin for 5 or 7 days. Ceftriaxone injections for either 5 or 10 days were compared in a noninferiority trial by Leophonte and colleagues.[7] Another cephalosporin study by Siegel and colleagues[8] used an initial 2-day regimen of intravenous cefuroxime followed by either 5 or 8 days of oral cefuroxime therapy. And, the only macrolide study by Tellier and colleagues[9] compared telithromycin once daily for either 5 or 7 days. In all of these studies, the shorter duration regimens demonstrated equivocal results to the longer duration regimens.

There are also 3 human studies that compare different durations of therapy where the regimen is not identical. A large, multicenter study of pneumonia in ventilator-dependent intensive care patients by Chastre and colleagues[10] evaluated randomly assigned 8- and 15-day courses of therapy where the regimen was determined by the attending physician. In this study, the distribution of regimen inclusions in the 8- and 15-day groups was very similar. Another study by Schönwald and colleagues[11] evaluated the same total dose of azithromycin given over 3 or 5 days in cases of

Table 1
Summary of human pneumonia studies evaluating duration of therapy

Reference	Type of Pneumonia	Regimen Comparison	Outcome Time Points	Outcome Difference?
Alteration in dose only				
el Moussaoui et al,[5] 2006	Adults admitted to the hospital with mild to moderate-severe community-acquired pneumonia (121 patients)	Initial 3 d of intravenous amoxicillin; patients with satisfactory response to IV therapy were assigned either to placebo or 750 mg amoxicillin 3 times daily for 5 additional days	The primary outcome was test-of-cure at day 10 (2 d after cessation of either placebo or oral amoxicillin) with a test to exclude inferiority of the placebo with a 10% margin as the delta for inferiority testing	Discontinuing amoxicillin treatment after 3 d is not inferior to discontinuing after 8 d when there was substantial improvement after 3 d
File Jr et al,[6] 2007	Mild to moderate community-acquired pneumonia in 469 patients	Gemifloxacin once daily for 5 or 7 d	Noninferiority test of clinical resolution at the end of therapy (days 7–9) and follow-up (days 24–30) with a 10% delta	Gemifloxacin for 5 d was not inferior to a 7 d course in respect to clinical, bacteriologic, and radiologic efficacy
Leophonte et al,[7] 2002	Community-acquired pneumonia in 186 hospitalized patients	Ceftriaxone injections of 1 g for 5 or 10 d	Noninferiority test with 10% delta for primary criteria of apyrexia at day 10 without resorting to another antibiotic, also clinical normalization at day 10, clinical and radiologic cure at day 10, and absence of the need for another antibiotic by day 10	Equivalent efficacy for all parameters; success at day 10 was 81.9% and 82.6% for the 5- and 10-d groups, respectively; success rates out to days 30 and 45 were not different between groups
Siegel et al,[8] 1999	Moderately severe community-acquired pneumonia in 52 hospitalized patients	Initial therapy of intravenous cefuroxime 750 mg every 8 h for 2 d followed by either 5 or 8 d of oral therapy with 500 mg cefuroxime every 12 h	Follow-up period of 42 d	No differences in cure rate, 87.5% cure with 5 d and 90.9% with 8 d of continued therapy

(continued on next page)

Table 1
(continued)

Reference	Type of Pneumonia	Regimen Comparison	Outcome Time Points	Outcome Difference?
Tellier et al,[9] 2004	Community-acquired pneumonia in 320 patients	Telithromycin, 800 mg once daily for 5 or 7 d	Clinical cure at the post-therapy test-of-cure visit on days 17–21	No difference in outcome; clinical cure rates of 89.3% and 88.8%, and satisfactory bacteriologic outcome rates of 87.7% and 80.0%, for the 5 and 7 d courses, respectively
Alteration in both regimen and duration				
Chastre et al,[10] 2003	Culture-confirmed, ventilator-associated pneumonia in 401 intensive care adult patients who had received appropriate previous empirical therapy	Antibiotic regimen was up to the attending physician and might change based on culture characteristics; durations were set at either 8 or 15 d	Noninferiority for death from any cause and microbiologically documented pulmonary infection recurrence; and superiority of antibiotic-free days for the 8 d regimens with a delta of 10%, all assessed at 28 d after the first bronchoscopy for suspected pneumonia onset	No differences detected in mortality or recurrence; at 28 d, 18.8% of the 8 d group and 17.2% of the 15 d group had died; microbiologically documented pulmonary infection recurrence rate was 28.9% and 26% for 8 and 15 d, respectively; no differences among drugs used in both groups; there were significantly more antibiotic-free days in the 8-d compared with the 15-d group
Schönwald et al,[11] 1991	Patients with clinical and radiologic findings of atypical pneumonia; only patients with known causative pathogens were included	A total 1.5 g dose of azithromycin, either 500 mg/d for 3 d, or 250 mg twice on day 1 followed by 250 mg once daily for days 2–5	Cure established on day 5	All patients were clinically cured by day 5 with a total of 1.5 g azithromycin given in either manner
Shorr et al,[12] 2005	Community-acquired pneumonia in patients ≥65 y old	Levofloxacin 750 mg/d for 5 or 500 mg/d for 10 d	Clinical and microbiologic endpoints 7–14 d after the last dose	No difference in outcome success, 89.0% and 91.9% in the 5 and 10 d groups, respectively

atypical pneumonia with a confirmed pathogen. The fluoroquinolone study in this group was by Shorr and colleagues,[12] and evaluated levofloxacin at 750 mg/d for 5 days or 500 mg/d for 10 days. As for the previous 5 studies, all of the 3 studies with the added variation of regimen also found equivocal results between the shorter and longer durations of therapy.

Because these types of clinical data related to duration of therapy are lacking for BRD, perhaps the most useful application of the human data is to give incentive for evaluating shortened exposures as new regimens are evaluated. The original approval work for ceftiofur sodium (Ceftiofur, Zoetis) in treating cattle with BRD allowed cattle classified as not responding after 3 days of therapy to receive 2 additional days of therapy.[13] Animals receiving additional therapy resulted in a higher cure rate at day 5 than at day 3, but it is not possible to determine from the available data what proportion of the increased cure rate was owing to the additional therapy as opposed to the additional time allowed for recovery.

The lack of evidence for optimal duration of treatment is a ubiquitous problem, and not just relegated to BRD in veterinary medicine. For example, a recent review by Jessen and colleagues[14] demonstrated that there are no available data to drive decisions related to the optimal duration of therapy for canine urinary tract infections.

How long should antimicrobial exposure in BRD therapy persist to ensure the optimum balance between brevity of exposure and maximum number of successful treatments? The answer is that there are no studies providing clinical data to drive that decision. It is possible to hypothesize that the optimal duration is based on the duration of antimicrobial exposure needed to eliminate the infectious agent, or to suppress the infectious agent to a critical point where recovery based on the physiologic response of the animal is ensured. In addition, it is important to note that the antimicrobial is acting within the context of the immune response to infection. The fact that not all clinical cures are owing to the antimicrobial is well-illustrated in a recently published review of the contribution of antimicrobials to BRD clinical outcomes as demonstrated in negative control randomized clinical trials.[15] In these studies, negative control groups indicate that clinical resolution of BRD occurs without therapy even in high-risk cattle. If clinical cures can occur in the absence of antimicrobials, then a reasonable hypothesis is that continued improvement in BRD clinical status may occur after cessation of therapy in some cases without the continued presence of an antimicrobial. These considerations of cure and case improvement with and without attribution to an antimicrobial effect are obviously influenced heavily by the accuracy of our case definitions for both disease and cure.

DURATION OF THERAPY: HOW LONG IS IT?

Consideration of when the antimicrobial is able to and not able to contribute to clinical outcome has been based on concentration of the antimicrobial (pharmacokinetics) related to the amount of drug necessary to impede pathogenicity of the pathogen in the animal (pharmacodynamics). A surrogate indicator of when the pathogenicity of a pathogen is neutralized has been the ability of the antimicrobial to suppress growth in the laboratory, expressed as the minimal inhibitory concentration (MIC). The MIC has been compared with multiple types of measured concentrations in the target animal, and conclusions made as to when the measured concentration(s) fall below the MIC. Although these relationships are informative, it is important to note that an MIC is a laboratory indicator variable for a clinical outcome related to a specific regimen when a broad range of data have been considered. These data include MIC distribution in relation to the potential for the presence of resistance genes, MIC distribution in relation to clinical outcome, and pharmacokinetics/pharmacodynamics of the antimicrobial. For a review of antimicrobial susceptibility testing related to cattle, the reader is referred to reviews by Lubbers and by Lubbers and Turnidge.[16,17]

Frankly, pharmacokinetics/pharmacodynamics and MIC relationships may be misleading as a guide to the duration of antimicrobial effect because they may be based on the extrapolation of in vitro pharmacodynamics from other bacterial species under ideal laboratory conditions combined with the pharmacokinetic measurements of drug concentrations in multiple matrices. These drug concentrations may contain significant proportions of the measured drug that are not available to interact with the pathogen. This overestimation of drug effect may be owing to drug binding, inoculum effect of large bacterial populations, or local conditions at the site of infection (eg, oxygen tension, pH), all of which dramatically change the drug–pathogen interaction. An example of potential overestimation of an antimicrobial effect is lung homogenate concentrations of macrolides compared with pathogen MIC distributions, whereas plasma concentration of the macrolides compared with pathogen MICs likely greatly underestimate the potential effect.

In common clinical use for BRD therapy, a time of effect of 24 hours past the last administration has been classically assumed for antimicrobials requiring daily administration for BRD, such as ampicillin trihydrate, erythromycin, sulfadimethoxine, spectinomycin, 100 mg/mL oxytetracycline products, tylosin, and procaine penicillin G. This assumption has led to PTIs of 24 hours after the last administration, based on the assumption that if recovery has not occurred by this time, then further antimicrobial presence is necessary to facilitate eventual recovery.

There are also single injection antimicrobials for which PTI recommendations have not been constructed through clinical trials. In these cases, such as single-injection oxytetracycline products and florfenicol, evaluating plasma concentration profiles helps to establish an estimated duration of therapy effect, although with the caveats mentioned.

Oxytetracycline (200 mg/mL)

Pharmacokinetic data for 200 mg/mL single injection oxytetracycline products administered intramuscularly at the label single injection regimen of 20 mg/kg suggest that plasma concentrations are in the approximate ranges of 1.0, 0.2, and 0.1 µg/mL at 48, 72, and 96 hours, respectively.[18] Subcutaneous administration would be expected to display similar pharmacokinetics. Establishment of a reasonable MIC target may be based on published surveillance data; a 10-year surveillance of MIC distributions for *Mannheimia haemolytica* by Portis and colleagues[19] found that approximately 50% of the isolates had an MIC of 1 µg/mL or less, depending on the year. Taking the plasma concentration to MIC relationship as the most optimistic prediction, a postadministration effective concentration based on maintaining the plasma concentration above the pathogen MIC for susceptible isolates would be 48 hours. In the authors' experience, 72 hours of clinical effect is often assumed for 200 mg/mL oxytetracycline products, with success/failure decisions for BRD made at 72 or 96 hours after administration.

Florfenicol

When administered at 40 mg/kg subcutaneously, florfenicol displayed a maximum concentration of 6 µg/mL at 3 hours after administration with a 27-hour elimination half-time.[20] Approximate concentrations in the plasma, based on this concentration decay, would be 3 µg/mL at 30 hours, 1.5 µg/mL at 57 hours, 0.75 µg/mL at 84 hours (approximately 3.5 days), and 0.33 µg/mL at 108 hours. The *M haemolytica* MIC data reported by Portis and colleagues demonstrated approximately 80% of the isolates at an MIC of 0.5 μg/mL or less. Based on maintaining plasma concentration above this MIC for the pathogen, a 4-day therapy duration is reasonable to assume for susceptible isolates.

Enrofloxacin

A single injection of enrofloxacin has a relatively brief period of effect. However, the efficacy of this class of antimicrobial is based on total exposure of the drug to the pathogen as indicated by the area under the concentration curve, meaning that the exposure can be high and brief for clinical efficacy. After a single subcutaneous injection, combined unbound concentrations of enrofloxacin and ciprofloxacin are below the MIC for 90% of *M haemolytica* isolates in plasma and tissue fluid by 48 hours.[21] Although at first this might indicate that cattle should be evaluated for clinical success or failure at 48 to 72 hours, a study discussed elsewhere in this article regarding PTIs suggests that, for this drug class, the pharmacokinetics may not be the primary driver determining the most appropriate PTI estimates of duration of therapy, as discussed, and may not be entirely valid if it is considered that the efficacy of therapy may be related more closely to overall drug exposure and not the need to maintain the drug above the MIC of the pathogen. However, when the question is when it might be expected for the drug to still be contributing to clinical response, plasma or serum concentrations are informative. Clinical resolution may or may not depend on continuing drug concentrations in the case of BRD.

Other Bovine Respiratory Disease Antimicrobials

For drugs with prolonged plasma concentration profiles and pharmacodynamics based on shorter dosing intervals (eg, β-lactams such as ceftiofur), or major questions as to which concentrations should be compared with pathogen MICs (eg, macrolides such as tilmicosin and tulathromycin), the most informative data are from studies that actually evaluate different PTIs. This may also be true for antimicrobials such as the fluoroquinolones, where plasma duration may be of sufficiently short duration that the drug is largely eliminated before the animal has a chance to recover physiologically and appear as a clinical success. For these reasons, the author prefers the term "single injection" to "long-acting" because the overall effect of prolonged, lower drug concentrations at the tails of these regimens on clinical outcome would be very difficult to confirm as opposed to the additional time allowed for recovery in these regimens.

CLINICAL TRIAL EVALUATION OF POSTTREATMENT INTERVALS FOR SINGLE INJECTION ANTIMICROBIALS

PTIs for several of the treatment options for BRD in North America have been evaluated within a selected range of PTIs. Trial data are available evaluating PTIs for ceftiofur crystalline free acid, tulathromycin, and tilmicosin. An additional study comparing enrofloxacin with tulathromycin using a 7-day PTI for both drugs has also been conducted. All of the studies evaluating PTIs discussed here are from company reports, not from the peer-reviewed literature.

Ceftiofur Crystalline Free Acid

Three feedlots participated in a study to evaluate PTIs for ceftiofur crystalline free acid.[22] When cattle were removed from the home pen for clinical signs of BRD (abnormal respiration and depression), and had a rectal temperature of 104.0°F or greater (≥40°C), they were treated with ceftiofur crystalline free acid (Excede, Zoetis) according to label directions. The treated cattle were randomly allocated to PTIs of 3,

5, or 7 days and were not eligible for further therapy until the PTI had passed. A summary of results are presented in **Table 2**. No differences were found in treatment success rates at the first day of eligibility after PTI for each group (a range of 92.9% to 96.3%). However, a significant difference between 28-day treatment success rates were found between the 3-day PTI group and the 7-day PTI group, at 65.5% and 77.5%, respectively. No differences were found in overall mortality rate or average daily gain through day 28.

These findings were supported by another study, which demonstrated significantly improved day 56 treatment success for a 7-day PTI as opposed to a 3-day PTI for ceftiofur crystalline free acid.[23] The 3-day PTI success rate in this study was similar to a 3-day PTI for enrofloxacin, but no 7-day PTI enrofloxacin group was included for comparison to the 7-day PTI ceftiofur crystalline free acid treatment group.

Tulathromycin

The original approval data for tulathromycin (Draxxin, Zoetis) evaluated clinical success at 14 days after treatment, but cattle could be classified as a failure and removed from the study for further treatment on study days 3 to 13 if failure criteria were met.[24] In subsequent tulathromycin studies, PTIs of 7, 10, and 14 days were evaluated where cattle were not eligible for further treatment until the designated PTI.[25] These studies used crossbred heifer feeder calves with a mean body weight of 215 kg (range, 147–291) originating from Missouri, Arkansas, Kentucky, and Tennessee. Entrance into the study required a combination of a clinical condition score of 1, 2, or 3 on a scale of 0 to 4, combined with a rectal temperature 104.0°F or greater ($\geq 40°C$). Cattle meeting entrance criteria were randomly assigned to either a 7-, 10-, or 14-day PTI before they were eligible for further treatment. The results of the study are summarized in **Table 3**. There were no differences in outcomes between the 3 PTI groups, including treatment success, respiratory disease-associated mortality, or average daily gain.

Tilmicosin

Crossbred steer calves weighing from 183 to 321 kg from Colorado, Kansas, Oklahoma, and Wyoming were enrolled in a 28-day study conducted in Wellington, Colorado. Animals with a clinical score of 2 or higher on a scale of 1 to 5 combined with a

Table 2
Summary of ceftiofur crystalline free acid posttreatment interval (PTI) study

	3-d PTI	5-d PTI	7-d PTI
PTI + 1 day treatment success rate (%)[1]	94.1[a] (n = 254)	92.9[a] (n = 255)	96.3[a] (n = 256)
28-d treatment success rate (%)[2]	65.5[a] (n = 253)	73.8[a,b] (n = 251)	77.5[b] (n = 255)
Retreatment success rate > day 9 (%)[3]	60.1[a] (n = 48)	59.9[a] (n = 33)	69.0[a] (n = 17)
Mortality owing to BRD (%)	1.57	1.57	1.17
ADG through 28 d (lb/d)[4]	2.93[a] (n = 256)	2.91[a] (n = 247)	2.85[a] (n = 251)

Abbreviations: ADG, average daily gain; BRD, bovine respiratory disease.

[a,b] Values in a row with different superscripts are statistically different ($P<.05$).

[1] Percentage of cattle that did not qualify for retreatment on the first day they were eligible (the first day after the PTI).

[2] Percentage of cattle that never qualified for retreatment during the study.

[3] Percentage of cattle that were retreated between the first day they were eligible, but before day 9, and never qualified for additional treatment during the study.

[4] Dead and other animals removed from the study were not included in the analysis.

Table 3
Summary of tulathromycin posttreatment interval (PTI) study

	7 d PTI	10 d PTI	14 d PTI
Animals enrolled	253	253	253
Removals (non-BRD or protocol deviation)[a]	5	2	3
Treatment success % (n)	85.9 (213/248)	85.3 (214/251)	88.8 (222/250)
BRD mortality % (n)	0.8 (2/248)	0.8 (2/251)	0.4 (1/250)
First nonresponse	23	31	23
Second nonresponse	7	4	3
Third nonresponse	2	0	0
BRD chronics % (#)	0.4 (1/248)	0 (0/251)	0.4 (1/250)
LSM average daily gain, deads out lb/d [SD] (range)	2.70 [0.70] (−0.18 to 4.14)	2.72 [0.67] (0.64–4.46)	2.55 [0.74] (−0.79 to 4.14)

Abbreviations: BRD, bovine respiratory disease; CNS, central nervous system; LSM, least square means.
[a] The 7-day group = 5 removals (2 CNS, 1 musculoskeletal, 1 traumatic reticuloperitonitis, 1 protocol deviation), 10-day group = 2 removals (1 protocol deviation, 1 abdominal disease), 14-day group = 3 removals (1 CNS, 2 musculoskeletal).

rectal temperature of 104.0°F or higher (≥40°C) were admitted to the study and treated with tilmicosin phosphate (Micotil, Elanco Animal Health) according to label directions. Cattle were assigned randomly to treatment groups consisting of 3-, 5-, or 7-day PTIs. As summarized in **Table 4**, the 28-day treatment success rate for a 7-day PTI was significantly greater than a 3-day PTI, with success rates of 86.9% and 67.9%, respectively. Treatment failures were determined at the time of conclusion of the PTI, and were not different, at 12.6%, 14.5%, and 8.1% for the 3-, 5-, and 7-day PTIs, respectively. Although only achieving a *P* value of .12 (most likely owing to limited numbers as compared with successes), it seems the main difference was the relapse percentages (initially categorized as a treatment success, then treated again at a later date), at 19.6%, 12.5%, and 5.0%, for the 3-, 5-, and 7-day PTIs, respectively.

Enrofloxacin

Although there is not an available study that evaluates different PTIs for enrofloxacin (Baytril, Bayer) there is a study of interest for comparing a 7-day PTI for both

Table 4
Summary of tilmicosin posttreatment interval study

Moratorium Length	3 d	5 d	7 d	Overall *P* Value
Number of pens	10	10	10	—
Number head	97	96	98	—
First treatment success (%)	67.9[a]	73.0[a,b]	86.9[b]	.05
Treatment failure (%)	12.6	14.5	8.1	.54
Relapse (%)	19.6	12.5	5.0	.12
Second relapse (%)	9.3[a]	1.0[b]	0.0[b]	.01
New episodes	2.1	4	1.1	.62
Day 0–56 BRD mortality (%)	2	3	0	.39

Abbreviation: BRD, bovine respiratory disease.
[a,b] Values in a row with different superscripts are statistically different (*P*<.05).

enrofloxacin and tulathromycin in the same study.[26] High-risk heifer calves weighing 161 to 305 kg were treated for control of respiratory disease on arrival with an observed interval of 3 days until the heifers were eligible for meeting treatment criteria. When treatment criteria were met, the heifers were allocated randomly to either tulathromycin or enrofloxacin administered as single subcutaneous injections of 2.5 mg/kg of tulathromycin and 12.5 mg/kg of enrofloxacin. Treatment success at the end of the 7-day PTI was the same for both groups at 85%. The overall treatment success at the end of the 28-day study was 55.5% (55/99) for tulathromycin and 48% for enrofloxacin (48/100). A χ^2 analysis by this author on the 28-day success rates resulted in a P value of .33, indicating that the 28-day outcome was not different among these treatments.

Data are needed that compare different PTIs for enrofloxacin to make definitive conclusions as to the effect of PTI duration. However, this study suggests that such a study would be useful to consider the effect of PTI in the case of an antimicrobial, which is not dependent on prolonged durations of concentrations above the MIC.

DISCUSSION

Data are not available to drive a definitive conclusion on the duration of drug exposure for therapy of BRD that will optimize efficacy while minimizing selection for resistant pathogens. Studies investigating therapeutic durations for human pneumonia consistently show that shorter durations of therapy may be equivocal, if not advisable. Although the multiple differences between human and BRD are recognized, it is reasonable to at least consider that these data encourage evaluation of shorter term exposures when possible.

Pharmacokinetic studies evaluated in light of pharmacodynamics of antimicrobials used for therapy of BRD may be informative as to when the antimicrobial is no longer able to contribute to continued recovery if the pathogen has not been inhibited sufficiently or eliminated. The concept of a PTI has evolved initially in concert with this concept of duration of therapy. In essence, prolonged PTIs were initially investigated based on estimations of when the drug is no longer able to contribute to treatment success, and therefore the animal would require additional therapy if clinical success has not been achieved. However, some clinical data support the concept that duration of drug concentrations in various matrices may not necessarily be the primary driver of the optimal PTI; examples are studies related to tilmicosin and enrofloxacin.

Clinical data comparing different PTIs for a fixed regimen are the ultimate source for informing our PTI decisions. Even then, these observations are confounded by the difference in time from when an animal is assured of eventual clinical success and when a qualified observer would use their observations along with quantitative data (eg, rectal temperature) to classify an animal as a clinical success. In mild or very acute cases, the clinical appearance may reflect immediately that the animal will be a treatment success. However, in more severe disease challenges, or when the animal is also undergoing other concurrent stressors, the success of the antimicrobial may not be evident until the physiologic state of the animal returns toward a normal state.

Regardless of various hypothesis as to the reasons for outcomes in the PTI studies cited here, there seems to be a pattern supporting a PTI of at least 7 days across multiple antimicrobial pharmacokinetic presentations. For tulathromycin, the study presented shows neither an advantage nor a disadvantage for extending the PTI beyond 7 days. The optimal PTI for ceftiofur crystalline free acid was 7 days, the longest PTI evaluated. In the case of tilmicosin, extending to a 7-day PTI resulted in a higher success rate than a 3- or 5-day PTI. Enrofloxacin performed similarly to tulathromycin when both drugs were allowed a 7-day PTI, despite pharmacokinetics that suggest that animals not responding to enrofloxacin by 3 days would not have additional drug effect to aid in further recovery.

This author's opinion is that the success of prolonged PTIs may be as much owing to giving the animal additional time to allow for clinical indices to match the clinical outcome as being due to a continued effect of drug concentrations in allowing the animal to finally become "cured." In other words, perhaps the prolonged presence of lesser concentrations of the drug may have given us the courage to wait longer for the animal's clinical indicators to match what would have been their eventual outcome regardless of drug presence or absence.

A challenge to prolonged PTIs has been that animals with a poor clinical appearance early or at a midpoint in the PTI cause great concern to animal care personnel, and the wisdom of not providing immediate additional therapy is questioned. An examination of the eventual outcomes of animals that display prolonged clinical signs during the PTI across multiple studies would be of great benefit; studies tend to just report overall success rate, and also don't report the number of animals displaying prolonged clinical sign resolution during the PTI, which are then declared a success at the end of the PTI.

Both the ceftiofur crystalline free acid and the tilmicosin PTI studies suggest that the difference in overall treatment success with the 7-day PTI may be owing to fewer relapses after the animals were declared an initial success. If initial treatment success is similar, then why would waiting for an additional period result in less relapses after a similar initial treatment success? One hypothesis may be related to additional time for recovery before subjecting the animal to handling and additional examinations. Regardless of the reasons, the industry would greatly benefit from additional research related to optimizing PTIs.

SUMMARY

Overall, the industry is making great advances in understanding the application of PTIs. As the struggle continues to select the optimal duration of therapy which maximizes clinical efficacy while minimizing selection for resistant respiratory pathogens, understanding when to apply success/failure criteria will be a critical component.

REFERENCES

1. Lubbers BV, Hanzlicek GA. Antimicrobial multidrug resistance and coresistance patterns of *Mannheimia haemolytica* isolated from bovine respiratory disease cases–a three-year (2009–2011) retrospective analysis. J Vet Diagn Invest 2013;25(3):413–7.
2. Pinzone MR, Cacopardo B, Abbo L, et al. Duration of antimicrobial therapy in community acquired pneumonia: less is more. ScientificWorldJournal 2014; 2014:759138.
3. Aliberti S, Giuliani F, Ramirez J, et al. How to choose the duration of antibiotic therapy in patients with pneumonia. Curr Opin Infect Dis 2015;28(2):177–84.
4. Pugh R, Grant C, Cooke RP, et al. Short-course versus prolonged-course antibiotic therapy for hospital-acquired pneumonia in critically ill adults. Cochrane Database Syst Rev 2011;(10):CD007577.
5. el Moussaoui R, de Borgie CA, van den Broek P, et al. Effectiveness of discontinuing antibiotic treatment after three days versus eight days in mild to moderate-severe community acquired pneumonia: randomised, double blind study. BMJ 2006;332(7554):1355.

6. File TM Jr, Mandell LA, Tillotson G, et al. Gemifloxacin once daily for 5 days versus 7 days for the treatment of community-acquired pneumonia: a randomized, multicentre, double-blind study. J Antimicrob Chemother 2007;60(1):112–20.
7. Leophonte P, Choutet P, Gaillat J, et al. Efficacy of a ten day course of ceftriaxone compared to a shortened five day course in the treatment of community-acquired pneumonia in hospitalized adults with risk factors. Med Mal Infect 2002;32(7): 369–81.
8. Siegel RE, Alicea M, Lee A, et al. Comparison of 7 versus 10 days of antibiotic therapy for hospitalized patients with uncomplicated community-acquired pneumonia: a prospective, randomized, double-blind study. Am J Ther 1999;6(4): 217–22.
9. Tellier G, Niederman MS, Nusrat R, et al. Clinical and bacteriological efficacy and safety of 5 and 7 day regimens of telithromycin once daily compared with a 10 day regimen of clarithromycin twice daily in patients with mild to moderate community-acquired pneumonia. J Antimicrob Chemother 2004;54(2):515–23.
10. Chastre J, Wolff M, Fagon JY, et al. Comparison of 8 vs 15 days of antibiotic therapy for ventilator-associated pneumonia in adults: a randomized trial. JAMA 2003;290(19):2588–98.
11. Schönwald S, Skerk V, Petricevic I, et al. Comparison of three-day and five-day courses of azithromycin in the treatment of atypical pneumonia. Eur J Clin Microbiol Infect Dis 1991;10(10):877–80.
12. Shorr AF, Zadeikis N, Xiang JX, et al. A multicenter, randomized, double-blind, retrospective comparison of 5- and 10-day regimens of levofloxacin in a subgroup of patients aged > or =65 years with community-acquired pneumonia. Clin Ther 2005;27(8):1251–9.
13. FDA/CVM. Food and drug administration FOIA drug summaries NADA 140–338 naxcel sterile powder - original approval. Rockville (MD): Food and Drug Administration Center for Veterinary Medicine; 1988. Available at: http://www.fda.gov/AnimalVeterinary/Products/ApprovedAnimalDrugProducts/FOIADrugSummaries/ucm049764.htm.
14. Jessen LR, Sorensen TM, Bjornvad CR, et al. Effect of antibiotic treatment in canine and feline urinary tract infections: a systematic review. Vet J 2015; 203(3):270–7.
15. DeDonder KD, Apley MD. A review of the expected effects of antimicrobials in bovine respiratory disease treatment and control using outcomes from published randomized clinical trials with negative controls. Vet Clin North Am Food Anim Pract 2015;31(1):97–111, vi.
16. Lubbers B. Using individual animal susceptibility test results in bovine practice. Vet Clin North Am Food Anim Pract 2015;31(1):163–74, vii.
17. Lubbers BV, Turnidge J. Antimicrobial susceptibility testing for bovine respiratory disease: getting more from diagnostic results. Vet J 2015;203(2):149–54.
18. Craigmill AL, Holland RE, Robinson D, et al. Serum pharmacokinetics of oxytetracycline in sheep and calves and tissue residues in sheep following a single intramuscular injection of a long-acting preparation. J Vet Pharmacol Ther 2000;23(6):345–52.
19. Portis E, Lindeman C, Johansen L, et al. A ten-year (2000–2009) study of antimicrobial susceptibility of bacteria that cause bovine respiratory disease complex—*Mannheimia haemolytica*, *Pasteurella multocida*, and *Histophilus somni*—in the United States and Canada. J Vet Diagn Invest 2012;24(5):932–44.
20. Sidhu P, Rassouli A, Illambas J, et al. Pharmacokinetic-pharmacodynamic integration and modelling of florfenicol in calves. J Vet Pharmacol Ther 2014;37(3):231–42.

21. Davis JL, Foster DM, Papich MG. Pharmacokinetics and tissue distribution of enrofloxacin and its active metabolite ciprofloxacin in calves. J Vet Pharmacol Ther 2007;30(6):564–71.
22. Outcomes of 3–, 5-, or 7-day post-treatment intervals after a single administration of EXCEDE. Technical Bulletin No. EXD04023. New York: Pfizer Animal Health; 2004.
23. Efficacy of excede followed by 3- or 7- day post-treatment intervals vs Baytril followed by a 3-day post-treatment interval in treatment of bovine respiratory disease. Technical Bulletin No. EXD04024. New York: Pfizer Animal Health; 2004.
24. Pfizer. Freedom of Information Summary new animal drug application 141-244 Draxxin injectable solution. Food and Drug Administration Center for Veterinary Medicine Freedom of Information Act Summaries. 2005. Available at: http://www.fda.gov/downloads/AnimalVeterinary/Products/ApprovedAnimalDrugProducts/FOIADrugSummaries/ucm118061.pdf. Accessed May 5, 2015.
25. Pfizer. Pfizer Animal Health Technical Bulletin. Efficacy of Draxxin, followed by 7-, 10–, or 14-day post-treatment intervals, against naturally occurring bovine respiratory disease. Prepared from study report 1133R-60-05-489. 2006.
26. Bayer. Field Trial Report 151.875. A comparison of the efficacy of Baytril 100 (enrofloxacin) and Draxxin (tulathromycin) for the treatment of bovine respiratory disease in feedlot cattle previously treated methaphylactically with Micotil (tilmicosin) upon arrival at the feedlot. 2006.

Management of Feedyard Hospitals

J.T. Fox, DVM, MS, PhD

KEYWORDS

- Cattle • Feedyard • Hospital • Husbandry

KEY POINTS

- Many types of hospital systems exist in commercial feedyards.
- The type of hospital system used must fit the facility design, the type of cattle fed at the feedyard, the crew that is employed by the feedyard, and the protocol established by the veterinarian.
- Managing animal inventory is critical throughout the convalescent phase.
- Animal husbandry is as important as the therapeutic plan.

INTRODUCTION

Little published data are available on best management practices for feedyard hospitals. This article addresses some of the common issues observed in the practice of feedyard medicine and provides related information on applicable topics. The goal here is to provide an unbiased view of options and issues surrounding the management of hospitals and hospital cattle in a feedyard.

TYPES OF HOSPITAL PENS

In general, there are three major types of hospital pens on feedyards depending on what type of hospital system is used: (1) pens that contain recently treated cattle (hospital pen), (2) pens that contain cattle that have received the maximum number of treatments and will not be administered additional therapy (chronic/railer pen), and (3) pens that allow segregation of animals affected with buller steer syndrome (buller pen). Some facilities may also use extended-recovery pens for cattle that fit in a chronic/railer pen, and this system may benefit cattle through additional days in an environment with less competition for feed and water resources. Buller pens are necessary to isolate these animals unless alternative management tactics are used

The author has nothing to disclose.
Veterinary Research and Consulting Services, LLC, Hays, KS 67601, USA
E-mail address: foxbeefvet@gmail.com

to ensure the welfare of these animals, such as buller cages (structure made of pipe that physically impedes an animal from mounting the buller syndrome steer). The detriment of establishing too many hospital pens is the reduction in yard capacity that could be used for normal feeding pens. To ensure the safety of the food supply, medical-hold pens may also be established. These pens allow the feedyard to place cattle under lock and key when they are under meat withhold as a result of drug administration. Cattle are locked into these pens on the day of and often days preceding the shipment of their pen to harvest. This ensures there are no errors made or breakdown in communication within the facility that could put the food supply at risk. Some facilities choose to keep treated cattle in traditional hospital pens the entire time they are under meat withhold. This can make it difficult to manage the inventory of these cattle, but may be the best option in some situations.

TYPES OF HOSPITAL SYSTEMS

Treat and go-home systems reduce the need for multiple hospital pens in feedyards that feed a variety of types and sizes of cattle (ie, Holstein steers, high-risk calves, and heavy yearlings) are able to keep these populations segregated to alleviate issues with competition and other social stressors, and maximize response (**Fig. 1, Table 1**). The pitfall of this system is that it does not allow cattle time to consume feed or hay, and water; however, it does ensure that the animal does not miss a ration transition in their home pen. If an animal stays in the hospital for several days, recovers, then goes back to its home pen after being anorexic for multiple days, the last thing that animal needs is to overconsume a ration that is higher in starch than its rumen is adapted to digest. This abrupt change could induce a bout of acidosis and possible recrudescence of the original disease process.

Feedyards with very few hospitals that require moving cattle a considerable distance from the home pen to and from the hospital may not be the best situation for a treat and go-home system because of the extra stress on the compromised animal. Facilities with hospitals on nearly every alley are the most ideal for the treat and go-home system. There are also derivations of the treat and go-home system that allow cattle to be returned the morning following therapy and/or allow for severely compromised cases to remain in a hospital pen.

Rotation systems were developed around how antimicrobials were administered in feedyards in the past. Short duration, daily treatments were required and therefore cattle needed to be brought through the hospital every day for their follow-up therapy. With longer-acting antimicrobials now available, there is no need to keep cattle in the hospital for treatments on Days 2 and 3. However, many believe there is merit to maintaining cattle in a more comfortable environment with closer access to water and feed. The other side of that argument is that these cattle are commingled and exposed to animals that may be shedding different organisms or types of organisms that can complicate the disease process.[1,2] For this system to work properly, the inventory of these pens must be managed to avoid overcrowding when the facility experiences high morbidity.

Durable cure systems require a lot of capacity in hospital pens because cattle are there for a prolonged period of time. This system in a feedyard that feeds cattle with high morbidity would be a failure simply because of the number of cattle that have to be housed in hospital pens and sorted each day to determine those healthy enough to return, and those that require additional therapy if eligible. Similar to the rotation system, durable cure systems allow cattle access to more space and less competition for feed and water. Giving animals the greatest opportunity to overcome

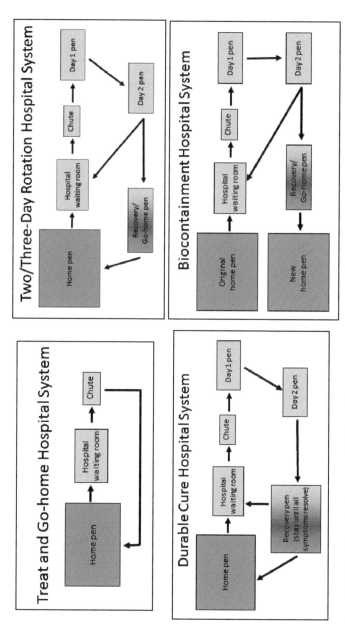

Fig. 1. Examples of feedyard hospital systems. (*Adapted from* Thomson D, Apley M. Hospital management in the commercial feedyard. Class in advanced feedlot production medicine. Kansas State University, College of Veterinary Medicine, Manhattan, KS; 2009.)

Table 1
Comparison of different types of hospital systems

Type	Pens Needed	Pros/Cons
Treat and go home	• Holding pen • Buller pen	Pros • Few pens to maintain • Easy cattle inventory management • No commingling of new cattle with late-day cattle (competition, disease exposure) • Does not detract from feed calls in home pen • During diet transitions, hospital cattle do not skip steps • Synergistic with longer (5+ day) posttreatment intervals Cons • No time allowed for recovery • Posttreatment intervals must be well-marked and followed by the staff because cattle are placed back in the home pen, and although not eligible for retreatment, they may still be showing clinical signs immediately after treatment • Competition for feed and water in home pen is often greater than in hospital pens • If an animal is affected with a metabolic disorder, they would not receive a break from a high-starch diet, or receive long-stem hay to stimulate salivation and rumen buffering
2- to 3-day rotation	• Day 1 pen • Day 2 pen • Recovery/go-home pen • Buller pen	Pros • Cattle stay in the hospital and have ample opportunity to consume hay and feed in a low-competition environment • Time for cattle to rest and regain strength before the return trip to home pen • Allows the crew to evaluate the animal for a few days before returning to the home pen Cons • More pens to manage and reduced feeding capacity of feedyard • Requires intense management of cattle inventories in computer software to ensure proper withdrawals are upheld, and home pens are fed proper amounts of feed because of the removal of the sick calves • Poor fit for treatments with a prolonged (>2 or 3 d) posttreatment interval • Becomes easy for crews to "lose" animals in the system (ie, they are not good enough to go back to their home pen, they are not bad enough to rail/realize, and these calves tend to accumulate in recovery/go-home pens if not well-managed)

(continued on next page)

Type	Pens Needed	Pros/Cons
Table 1 **(continued)**		
Durable cure	• Day 1 pen • Day 2 pen • Extended- recovery pen • Chronic pen • Buller pen	Pros • Benefits similar to the rotation system • The extended recovery may benefit unique cattle populations, such as lightweight naive calves, allowing them to recover in low-stress environment for a prolonged period and then "restart" back with the general population Cons • Pitfalls similar to the rotation system • Managing the accountability (who is responsible) for cattle in these pens can become challenging for the facility
Biocontainment	• Day 1 pen • Day 2 pen • New home pen • Chronic pen • Buller pen	Pros • Segregates all calves identified with disease from potential shedding back into initial cohort • Can be used for niche market programs, such as natural or organic, because it segregates animals that have received antimicrobial or steroid therapy, because these are commonly and/or always prohibited in these programs Cons • Cattle inventory management and accounting management becomes very complex with this system • Commingles all treated cattle from various home pens and origins that are experiencing various, and possibly unique disease processes in one new pen

disease and ship to harvest with their original cohort instead of being realized may be beneficial, but one must also consider the costs associated with maintaining these animals in a recovery facility for a prolonged period of time. There are obvious opportunity costs on these cattle when they could be replaced with a new arrival that is healthy, and grows faster and more efficiently.[3]

Biocontainment hospital systems may come in a variety of approaches, but the key item is that cattle meeting a certain case definition are not re-exposed to their original cohort. This system does have application with certain niche market programs where cattle that receive certain prespecified products, such as antimicrobials, are excluded from the program. By segregating at the time of administration it reduces the need to remove these animals from their original group at a later date. One major pitfall of this approach is that it commingles all of the clinical cases from the entire facility into one pen. The expected mortality on the new commingled group is relatively high compared with that of a traditional feeding group because it is equivalent to the case-fatality rate of the feedyard. It is likely advantageous to hold these cattle in the hospital pens (Days 1, 2, and recovery pens) for a few days before introducing to the new lot to allow recovery without competition, perhaps even holding until their post-treatment interval (PTI) has expired and they can be evaluated for additional therapy before introduction to the new pen.

MANAGING POST-TREATMENT INTERVALS

With the evolution of antimicrobial molecules and the application of evidence-based medicine, it is now known that by increasing the days before a second or third treatment the treatment response rate is improved in most cases. This period of time, referred to as a PTI, varies depending on the product used and perhaps even on the type of cattle in which it is used. This variability is what makes managing PTIs difficult. A feedyard employee must be able to recognize which animals are eligible for retreatment while simultaneously evaluating if it is necessary based on clinical evaluation. Maintaining a list of animal identification numbers that lists these dates may become quite cumbersome when working horseback. Actual marking of the animal using hide chalk or paint, writing dates on ear tags, or applying a temporary marking on the head of the animal are popular methods of conveying the end of the PTI for each individual (**Fig. 2**).

Newer technologies may allow an employee to scan an electronic tag with a hand-held device or smartphone and then be told whether or not that animal is under a PTI and additional information, such as when they were treated and what product was administered.

SORTING CATTLE IN THE HOSPITAL

Handling stress of treated cattle is inevitable because of the nature of separating and moving cattle from one location to another for therapy. However, through improved focus on training and auditing of cattle handling this situation has improved greatly throughout the industry and handlers should strive to continue to improve each and every day. When cattle are handled through the chute and administered their therapy, there is then the opportunity to sort or segregate them at this point to reduce the amount of handling subsequent to therapy. For instance, if a hospital is using a treat and go-home system and services three rows of pens, it is beneficial to sort the cattle three ways into their home alley as they receive therapy instead of having extra handling by sorting on foot or horseback when the cattle are returned to the home pens. Regardless of when cattle are sorted, handling them calmly and quietly is a must to reduce stress and maximize treatment response. Cattle that are severely compromised may have a heightened fight or flight response and can pose a safety hazard when handled by untrained individuals.

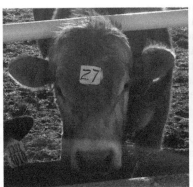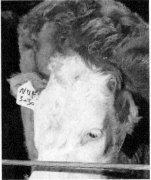

Fig. 2. Examples of marking cattle with their date of eligibility for retreatment following the posttreatment interval.

MANAGING ANIMAL INVENTORIES AND WITHHOLD TIMES

Most confined cattle operations use a software system to track animals on the facility. This includes where the each animal is currently located; what medicines have been administered to this animal; and, more importantly, when this animal is eligible to be sent to harvest based on meat withholding times. In many operations cattle are identified as a group or "lot" of animals that may or may not be representative of a separate pen where the animals are housed. This is because the same medicines are administered on arrival to all cattle and therefore the meat withhold time is the same for every individual. Cattle would then be identified individually when an individual treatment is administered and a unique meat withhold time is appreciated for that animal. Label directions of all medicines provide the number of days an animal must be withheld before becoming part of the food supply. Upholding these requirements is a pivotal role of all people at the feedyard because they are the front-line of defense to maintain the safety and security of the food supply. The problem with the software tracking is that it requires proper entry and updating for it to be correct.

For example, an animal identified as tag number 175 receives a treatment of interdigital phlegmon (more commonly called foot rot) and is entered in the computer as being in hospital pen C2. One employee from the feedyard returns this animal to his home pen, but does not enter or communicate this animal movement. This animal seems to be in hospital pen C2 in the software system, but is physically in his home pen. The errors that this can cause are numerous. If the home pen were to ship to harvest and animal 175 was under a meat withhold and is in the home pen, no one would know that they need to remove that animal before the pen is shipped. That is why it is a good practice to have a medicine-hold or hold-over pen and lock-up all cattle under withhold that belong to the lots of animals shipping on a given day. Additional issues with poor inventory management include improper headcounts for feeding purposes. The amount fed to a given pen of cattle is typically called based on an amount per number of cattle present. If the system lists the wrong number of cattle present it can yield less than perfect feed delivery amounts. Because of the concerns around inventory management and withhold times, some facilities may choose to leave cattle in hospital pens until they are clear of withhold. This may require large hospital pens depending on the facility and number of cattle treated.

HOSPITAL TANK AND PEN CLEANING

Cleanliness is the most basic form of animal husbandry. By reducing pathogen load, one reduces the draw on an animal's immune system and maximizes the response to therapy. The survival of bovine viral diarrhea virus in water with the provision of a mucus substrate was demonstrated to be 24% at 24 hours and 16% at 48 hours.[4] Cleaning these tanks on a daily basis removes this potential nidus and may also stimulate the cattle to drink. Alam and coworkers[2] found that cattle treated for respiratory disease have a very high prevalence of fecal shedding of Salmonella and depending on the specific strain, can have a significant impact on clinical outcome. The pens are often neglected from a pen cleaning standpoint because of the relatively low number of animals and manure accumulation, but based on pathogen concentration it is critical to improve the effectiveness of treatments. Many facilities provide bedding to these animals to alleviate cold stress in the winter and heat stress in the summer. A study evaluating bedding in dairies found that adding organic material, such as chopped straw, increased the moisture level and gram-negative pathogen content.[5] This stresses the importance of cleaning and removing bedding when it becomes wet to alleviate the additional pathogen load on these animals.

HOSPITAL FEED AND HAY PROVISION

Making appropriate feed calls (amounts) to hospital pens can be a complex process. This is because these cattle may have relatively low intakes because they are clinically ill and some are likely anorexic. To further complicate the situation, the headcount in these pens varies throughout the day based on animals moved to different pens and new animals being brought to the hospital. It is important that enough feed is provided for hospital cattle to consume without wasting feed that will not be eaten. Excess feed in these bunks should be removed every 2 to 3 days to ensure the feed is fresh and appealing and does not form mold in the feedbunk to detract cattle from wanting to eat. Rations that are higher in moisture (35% or higher) rapidly spoil in the bunk particularly in warmer times of the year.

The type of diet or ration fed to these pens can also require a lot of consideration. The most important consideration is that category II feed additives (those that require a meat withhold period) must be monitored if they are used in hospital pens because if animals are railed or realized the appropriate withhold must be upheld.[6] Furthermore, rations or batches of feed that are used to "flush" feed milling facilities or feed trucks after a type II feed additive must also be cautiously used in pens where cattle may be sent to harvest.

When deciding what ration to feed to a particular hospital pen, it is important to consider what the cattle in the hospital were being fed in their home pen and try to mimic that ration. Duff and Galyean[7] suggest that higher-concentrate diets fed as a receiving diet to high-stressed cattle may enhance proinflammatory cytokine and febrile response yielding longer periods of illness as noted by Lofgreen and collegues.[8] The provision of a grain-based concentrate in addition to hay actually yielded lower interferon production and a higher percent of animals shedding bovine rhinotracheitis virus at 9 days postchallenge compared with providing hay alone.[9] This suggests that providing hay alone may be a superior diet to maximize clinical response, but given that these cattle must return to their home feeding pens and eat high-concentrate diets it is critical to maintain and/or restore appropriate rumen microflora to digest these diets. Providing hay may have some benefit in animals that were incorrectly diagnosed as bovine respiratory disease and may actually be suffering from subacute or acute acidosis. Consuming hay forces the animal to spend more time chewing, which induces saliva production and buffers rumen pH. Hay can also serve as an attractant for cattle recovering from disease that may otherwise be anorexic. These animals may not be familiar with concrete feedbunks and concentrate-based diets and therefore providing a feedstuff the animal is more accustomed to may stimulate intake.

ADDITIONAL HUSBANDRY ITEMS

Shade has been well-documented to improve performance and ameliorate heat-stress.[10,11] Reducing heat stress in hospital pens is important considering the reduced pulmonary capacity in cattle with bovine respiratory disease.[12] Depending on the type of shade used, it may also offer protection from precipitation and cold stress during the colder months of the year. One consideration with shade is to ensure the conditions under the shade are well-kept so that this area does not become soaked with urine and feces, and actually create an environment that is worse than without the shade.

Windbreaks improve winter performance of cattle and suggest the impact of cold stress is at least partially mitigated by use of windbreaks.[13] These can, however, be counterproductive if they are a permanent structure that cannot be removed for the summer months.[13] These structures should not be completely solid, but allow 10% to 20% open space to allow them to work properly and to not create excessive drifting of snow.[13] If properly designed and maintained, shade and windbreak structures may provide additional improvements in animal comfort to reduce stress and improve response to therapy.

SUMMARY

There are many considerations when managing feedyard hospitals. The type of hospital system used must fit the facility design, the type of cattle fed at the feedyard, the crew that is employed by the feedyard, and the protocol established by the veterinarian. Ensuring the animals are well-cared for and have their basic needs met should be the priority of the feedyard personnel and the veterinarian maintaining the veterinarian-client-patient relationship with the feedyard.

REFERENCES

1. Briggs RE, Frank GH, Purdy CW, et al. Rapid spread of a unique strain of *Pasteurella haemolytica* serotype 1 among transported calves. Am J Vet Res 1998;59: 401–5.
2. Alam MJ, Renter DG, Ives SE, et al. Potential associations between fecal shedding of *Salmonella* in feedlot cattle treated for apparent respiratory disease and subsequent adverse health outcomes. Vet Res 2009;40:2.
3. Cernicchiaro N, White BJ, Renter DG, et al. Evaluation of economic and performance outcomes associated with the number of treatments after an initial diagnosis of bovine respiratory disease in commercial feeder cattle. Am J Vet Res 2013;74:300–9.
4. Stevens ET, Thomson DU, Wileman BW, et al. The survival of bovine viral diarrhea virus on materials. Bov Pract 2011;45:118–23.
5. Hogan JS, Smith KL, Hoblet KH, et al. Bacterial counts in bedding materials used on nine commercial dairies. J Dairy Sci 1989;72:250–8.
6. Food and Drug Administration. New animal drugs for use in animal feeds. CFR 2014; Title 21 6:558.3.
7. Duff GC, Galyean ML. Board-invited review: recent advances in management of highly stressed, newly received feedlot cattle. J Anim Sci 2007;85:823–40.
8. Lofgreen GP, El Tayeb AE, Kiesling HE. Millet and alfalfa hays alone and in combination with high-energy diets for receiving stressed calves. J Anim Sci 1981;52: 959–68.
9. d'Offay JM, Rosenquist BD. Combined effects of fasting and diet on interferon production and virus replication in calves infected with a vaccine strain of infectious bovine rhinotracheitis virus. Am J Vet Res 1988;49:1311–5.
10. Gaughan JB, Bonner S, Loxton I, et al. Effect of shade on body temperature and performance of feedlot steers. J Anim Sci 2010;88:4056–67.
11. Sullivan ML, Cawdell-Smith AJ, Mader TL, et al. Effect of shade area on performance and welfare of short-fed feedlot cattle. J Anim Sci 2011;89:2911–25.
12. Wittum TE, Woollen NE, Perino LJ, et al. Relationships among treatment for respiratory tract disease, pulmonary lesions evident at slaughter, and rate of weight gain in feedlot cattle. J Am Vet Med Assoc 1996;209:814–8.
13. Mader TL. Environmental stress in confined beef cattle. J Anim Sci 2003;81: E110–9.

Feedlot Euthanasia and Necropsy

Dee Griffin, DVM, MS

KEYWORDS

- Bovine • Euthanasia • Humane • Brain stem disruption (pithing) • Necropsy
- Diagnosis • Records

KEY POINTS

- Safety of the person euthanizing an animal, and other people in the vicinity, are the most critical considerations.
- Attempt to connect all necropsy observations to a unifying diagnosis.
- Use a necropsy data recording system that allows for analysis of linked necropsy findings across all production management considerations on an operation, across operations and/or regions.

FEEDLOT EUTHANASIA AND NECROPSY

This section includes:

- Euthanasia overview as can be practiced in beef feedlots
- A necropsy outline for feeder cattle that minimizes detached organs

FEEDLOT EUTHANASIA

The principal reason for considering euthanasia in a beef feedlot is to stop pain and suffering of cattle that have little chance of recovery or of pain abatement. As veterinarians, we have an ethical obligation and responsibility to ensure cattle are treated humanely. When warranted, euthanasia, meaning a "good death," must be considered.[1,2]

The feedlot's veterinarian should help management develop euthanasia SOPs (Standard Operating Procedures) BMP (Best Management Practice) appropriate for the feedlot. This will serve as a guide for identifying situations for which euthanasia should be considered and a guide for selecting the method(s) appropriate for the feedlot's safety concern. Additionally, the employee(s) training requirements should be listed and the employee(s) trained to administer the euthanasia technique must be

The author has nothing to disclose.
Great Plains Veterinary Educational Center, University of Nebraska – Lincoln, 820 Road 313, PO Box 148, Clay Center, NE 68933-0148, USA
E-mail address: DGRIFFIN@GPVEC.UNL.EDU

Vet Clin Food Anim 31 (2015) 465–482
http://dx.doi.org/10.1016/j.cvfa.2015.05.009
vetfood.theclinics.com

identified in the document. A copy of the euthanasia SOPs/BMP should be on file in the feedlot office. Euthanasia SOPs/BMP templates are available from the National Cattlemen's Beef Association Beef Quality Assurance Program and from the American Association of Bovine Practitioners.[3–5] These templates will provide a good starting place for developing a euthanasia SOPs/BMP that meets the needs of an individual feedlot. *Important note:* Cattle that will be rendered must not contain chemical residues that could be harmful to other animals that would consume rendered products.[6] The Food and Drug Administration (FDA) Center for Veterinary Medicine (CVM) regulates all animal feeds and the agency has not expressed a concern about rendered by-product contamination from cattle treated with FDA-CVM approved antimicrobials or approved adjunct therapy medications.

Conditions That Warrant Euthanasia Considerations

The following is a list of conditions that warrant euthanasia considerations[1,2]:

- Arthritis with multiple joints
- Central nervous system disorders
- Emaciation/dehydration
- Extreme lameness and reluctance to move
- Nonambulatory or unable to stand
- Peritonitis/pleuritis
- Pneumonia (unresponsive)
- Prolapsed uterus
- Ruptured bladder/uremia
- Septicemia/toxemia
- Severe anemia or jaundice
- Severe distress, for example following a severe injury
- Shock/imminent death
- Spinal injury
- Systemic neoplasia, extremely rare in feeder cattle

Euthanasia Intent, Considerations, and Safety

Although disagreement can arise about the method used to end an animal's life, generally there is unified acceptance that if the animal is to die, it must be a "good" death in that the animal should be handled in such a way as to minimize excitement, discomfort, and/or anxiety before being euthanized. The euthanizing technique should cause humane rapid loss of consciousness and subsequent death without evidence of pain or distress, or use anesthesia produced by an agent that causes painless loss of consciousness and subsequent death.[1,2]

The animal's well-being and the safety of humans and other animals in the vicinity of where the animal(s) will be euthanized must be the primary considerations. The 4 "S's" of safety must always be a primary concern. These are safety of yourself, safety of others working around you, safety of the animal, and safety of the food.[4]

Esthetically, humans seem to have less personal anxiety with the use of injectable euthanizing techniques than with firearms or captive bolts. However, the use of injectable euthanasia agents is more apt to cause apprehension and mental distress in cattle to be euthanized. The application of these agents requires some restraint and pain associated with the injection needle placement, which increases the level of anxiety. Additionally, there can be significant and serious consequences to improper disposal of cattle euthanized with injectable agents. The FDA forbids the use of barbiturates in cattle that are rendered for concern the barbiturate might cause harm in animal foods that use rendered product. Cattle euthanized with barbiturates must be buried, burned, or composted. Anyone one of these disposal techniques may require either Environmental Protection Agency or state Department of Environmental Quality permitting. Environmental half-life of barbiturates and the potential for scavenging by wild carnivores, raptors, and dogs loose in the community could come to serious peril if the euthanized animal(s) is/are not properly buried, burned, or composted.[1,2]

A potential alternative to barbiturate use in cattle would include the use of xylazine to induce deep sedation followed by an environmentally acceptable agent to disrupt vital organ function to cause quick death. Agents that are considered as the second injectable would include potassium chloride (KCl), magnesium sulfate (MgSO4) or a depolarizing muscle relaxant such as succinylcholine. NEVER USE ONE OF THESE AGENTS (KCL, MgSO4, or depolarizing muscle relaxants) TO CAUSE DEATH OF A CONSCIOUS ANIMAL! The same pragmatic statement might also be said of exsanguination. Unless the technique produces rapid exsanguination, such as at the skilled hands of a Rabbi, the animal should always be unconscious during the exsanguination procedure. Additionally, never use chemicals, such as quaternary ammonia, phenols, oxidizing agents, or other chemicals that have some other normal intended use that is not medical in nature.[1,2]

Captive Bolt and Gunshot Considerations

In many situations, the cattle's well-being would best be served if a firearm or captive bolt were used by a competent euthanasia technician to end the animal's life. Generally, animals will not recognize the instrument (firearm or captive bolt) and loss of consciousness should be instantaneous with the triggering of the devise. The safety of the technician and bystanders is paramount. Captive bolts require close approximation to the animal, which in some situations would be a safety hazard. Firearms could minimize the proximity concern, but safety of bystanders might be a serious issue in some situations. Esthetically, the noise and visual associated with a firearm or captive bolt may not be appropriate for some situations, such as euthanasia of an injured animal in public settings.[1,2]

A captive bolt can be dangerous to the operator if the targeted animal is not isolated, recumbent, and docile. An operator should never attempt to use a captive bolt on an animal when commingled within a group of cattle. Likewise, an operator should never attempt to use a captive bolt on an animal that is agitated until the animal can be brought under physical control. This is especially true in dealing with injured cattle remaining on a trailer.[4]

Sedative/Tranquilizer Use

A pole syringe is an excellent tool for delivering a sedative/tranquilizer to agitated cattle to quiet them, allowing a safe approach with a captive bolt. A pole syringe can be constructed using a small-diameter telescoping painter's pole that has had a washer attached to the end for accepting the black rubber seal from the plunger of a 60-mL disposable syringe. The painter's pole with attached 60-mL syringe becomes a tool for delivering a sedative/tranquilizer to the bovine. Note it is best to use the largest injection needle available, such as a 14 gauge 1.5 inch. Additionally, it is useful to use the plastic syringe case with a needle-size hole punched in the end to cover the syringe and needle. This covering will help prevent the injection needle from bending (**Fig. 1**).[4]

After the sedative takes effect, the animal can be safely approached with a captive bolt. The best sedative for this purpose is xylazine, as the effective dose for cattle is only a tenth the dose for other species, and it is denatured at 165°C and rendering temperatures are in excess of 240° C.[7,8]

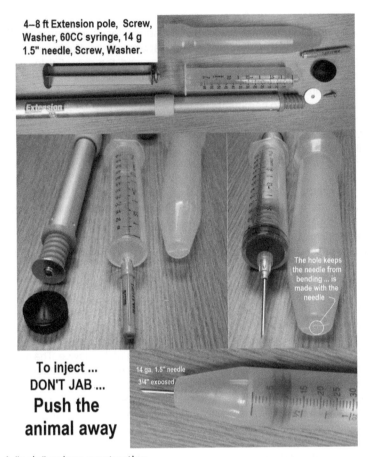

4–8 ft Extension pole, Screw, Washer, 60CC syringe, 14 g 1.5" needle, Screw, Washer.

Extension

The hole keeps the needle from bending ... is made with the needle

To inject ...
DON'T JAB ...
Push the animal away

14 ga, 1.5" needle
3/4" exposed

Fig. 1. A "pole" syringe construction.

Use of a Gun to Perform Euthanasia

Gunshot as a euthanasia technique for cattle is acceptable provided the shooter is trained in gun safety and is a qualified marksperson with the gun to be used and at the distance required for euthanizing the selected animal.[2–4] The first consideration, safety training should be conducted by an approved gun safety trainer. Typically there are classes offered in every community, and their times and locations can be obtained by contacting the local law enforcement office, university extension office, or gun store. From a liability standpoint, the feedlot's management should not take for granted an employee who says he or she is trained in safe gun handling has been properly trained and should have procedures for verifying their training and testing their knowledge and skill. Management should identify a select few employees who will be assigned the responsibility of using a gun for euthanizing cattle in the feedlot and those employees must obtain updated gun safety training. The training must include the type of gun that will be used on the feedlot. A copy of the training certificate for each employee so assigned should be on file in the feedlot office.[2,3]

Gun selection should consider the ballistics of the cartridge to be used and the aiming stability over the distance/range required to deliver the bullet to the vital targeted area on the animal. At least 350 ft-lb of ballistic energy is recommended for feeder cattle between 450 and 800 pounds and at least 500 ft-lb of ballistic energy is recommended for feeder cattle that weigh more than 800 pounds. **Table 1** lists the energy ballistics for different caliber cartridges and notes that all large-caliber rifles, shotgun slugs, and most large-caliber handguns provide sufficient ballistic energy for euthanizing feeder cattle. When safety is included in the selection, the distance that a bullet travels from a large-caliber rifle cartridge generally removes large-caliber rifles from consideration. Unless the distance from the gun to the euthanasia target on a bovine is short, handgun aiming accuracy is difficult. When bullet distance traveled and aiming accuracy is considered, a shotgun rifled slug is often the best choice for feedlot euthanasia considerations (see **Table 1**).[4]

Euthanasia Target Aiming

Generally, the brain is the target for a captive bolt or gunshot. On rare instances, a gunshot to the heart may need to be considered, but the heart as a target for euthanasia should never be considered first as a primary location (**Fig. 2**).[8] The landmarks for delivering a captive bolt stun or gunshot to the brain in cattle seem to be confusing. What one must know is the brain is above a line drawn across the animal's forehead at the level just above the eyes (**Fig. 3**). The boundary for this line is the location of the zygomatic arch meeting the frontal crest, typically, three-fourths to 1 inch above the

Table 1
Cartridge Ballistic Energy

Ballistics[a]	ft-lb
Small Handgun & Small Caliber Rifle	
22 Magnum	360
22 Hornet	733
Handgun (FMJ unless otherwise noted)	
9 MM	360
357 Magnum, SP (Soft Point)	537
40 SW (Smith & Wesson)	400
44 Magnum	741
45 ACP (Automatic Colt Pistol)	404
45 Colt, LRN (Lead Round Nose)	410
Large Caliber Rifle	
223 Remington	1099
243 Winchester	1819
270 Winchester	2754
308 Winchester	2800
30-06 Springfield	2997
30-30 Winchester	1611
7.62x39 FMJ (Full Metal Jacket) - SKS (Savez Komunista Srbije)	1653
Shotgun Rifled Slugs	
410 Gage Rifled Slug, 2.5"	654
410 Gage Rifled Slug, 3"	783
20 Gage Rifled Slug, 2.75"	1863
16 Gage Rifled Slug, 2.75"	1989
12 Gage Rifle Slug, 2.75"	2808

[a] Ballistics is the energy profile of ammunition measured in "Foot-Pounds" (ft-lb).

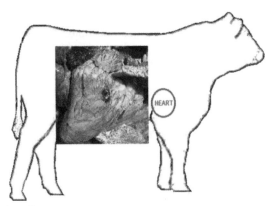

Fig. 2. Heart location diagram.

top of the eye. Note: This line is discussed later in this article as a landmark for brain removal during a necropsy. The location from both a front and side view is illustrated in **Fig. 4**. The tall, elongated pole on Holstein feeder cattle presents some targeting confusion, but as long as the lower brain landmark is considered, an effective gunshot or captive bolt placement is achieved.[2,4]

Secondary Technique Used to Ensure Death

Secondary techniques used to ensure death should be included following either captive bolt application or a gunshot.[1,2] Exsanguination is used daily around the world as part of a sequence of techniques used to produce humane death of cattle intended for human food. Exsanguination is a reliable secondary technique to ensure death of animals euthanized by gunshot or captive bolt. Intra-abdominal exsanguination by cutting the descending aorta with a scalpel through the rectal wall might be a useful technique for large animals as the second part of a euthanizing process that starts with the use of a medication that renders the animal unconscious. *Veterinarians and laymen should never use exsanguination as the only euthanizing technique in conscious animals*. The use of intravenous KCL or MgSO4 as a secondary step after captive bolt or gunshot is also acceptable. However, both of these cause rapid blood coagulation; therefore, it can be difficult to get sufficient quantity to get the desired result.[1,2]

Brains stem disruption (BSD), using a rigid small-diameter rod, is the most reliable and simplest secondary technique I have used following a captive bolt or cranial

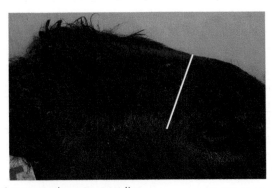

Fig. 3. Brain location, ventral-most extent line.

P = Top Front of Pole   Z = Zygomatic Arch Frontal Crest Junction

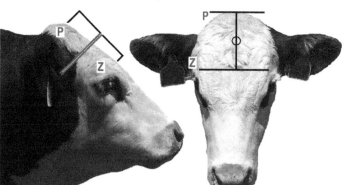

Fig. 4. Euthanasia captive bolt or gunshot aiming point. (*Data from* Gilliam JN, Shearer JK, Woods J, et al. Captive-bolt euthanasia of cattle: determination of optimal-shot placement and evaluation of the Cash Special Euthanizer Kit for euthanasia of cattle. Anim Welf 2012;21(4 Suppl 2):99–102.)

gunshot. It is far superior to any other secondary technique. The technique requires a small-diameter 15-inch length of stiff rod. A one-eighth-inch to one-quarter-inch welding filler rod works well. The rod is placed in the hole produced by the captive bolt or bullet and directed toward the foramen magnum (**Fig. 5**). There will be a slight stiffening of the animal's legs as the rod reaches the brain stem.[4]

FEEDLOT NECROPSY

When asked, "What is the purpose of a necropsy?" the answer is invariably, "To determine the cause of death." In a feedlot generally, that is not the case. Most cattle that

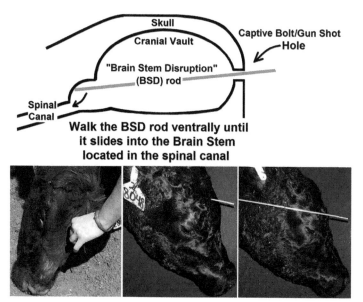

Fig. 5. BSD rod use diagram series.

die in feedlot settings have sufficient history and circumstantial information surrounding their death to, with some accuracy, predict the "cause of death." I have 2 reasons for doing feedlot necropsies. First, it is a little like opening a Christmas present, you never know for sure what you are going to find. Second, and the principal reason for doing a necropsy, is to, with some accuracy, assign the animal cause of death to a management area in a feedlot. The management areas include cattle acquisition, arrival processing, sickness observation, treatment protocols, feed management, and facilities maintenance.[4]

Each of management areas considered when doing a feedlot necropsy has subareas to consider. For example, cattle acquisition should consider source in terms of distance hauled, likelihood of cattle coming from herds in which a health management plan is followed, particular diseases common to an area (eg, flukes, parasite hypobiosis), and previous health issues from previous cattle from a source or geographic area. Examples for feed management may include subclinical acidosis, foreign bodies, particle size–associated bloat, and 3-methylindole–associated atypical interstitial pneumonia (AIP). Clinical AIP is a great example supporting the reason to do feedlot necropsies, as the syndrome can be related to feed management or a sequela from a previous pneumonia. Grossly, finding visual evidence of edema and emphysema along with evidence of a previous pneumonia, pushes this death into the health management group rather than the feed management group. Histologically, these are often diagnosed as alveolar or bronchial obstructions.[4]

Because gaining information that may be used to evaluate production or influence production management decisions is key and because many production management issues are interrelated, doing a complete and thorough assessment of organ systems is critical to draw meaningful conclusions. My approach is one learned from the US Department of Agriculture Food Safety Inspection Service (FSIS). The FSIS abattoir inspection system focuses on inspecting organ system–associated lymph nodes (**Fig. 6**). If the lymph nodes draining a body system are normal, there typically is no reason to perform a detailed examination of the body system beyond a general visual

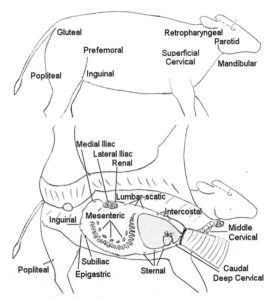

Fig. 6. Bovine lymph node location diagram.

overview. There are exceptions in which associated lymph nodes do not indicate the problem, such as the central nervous system (CNS), heart, lungs, and joints. Examining the lung-associated lymph nodes is extremely useful as an adjunct observation for assessing acuteness, activeness, and chronicity of other visual gross lung tissue observations. Another example is the tipoff provided by the hepatic lymph node that liver flukes may be present when black discoloration is observed.[4]

Necropsy Safety, Tools, and Technique

Safety is the first priority. Protective clothing, gloves, and boots that can be disinfected are a must. Remind everyone around to be careful to prevent or at least minimize their personal contamination. Adequate supplies should be present to adequately clean tools and equipment after the procedure.

Sharp Knives Are a Must!

A "V" carbide blade knife sharpener is a quick alternative to using a knife-sharpening abrasive. Although the edge is very course, it is a usable edge on a necropsy knife blade.

Sharpening knives

Diamond-coated steel slabs are more durable than stone abrasives. They are easily cleaned and having an assortment of different grits is useful. Holding the blade at a consistent angle during sharpening is critical. There are several diamond-coated sharpening abrasives designed to maintain a consistent sharpening angle. Most have a clamp to hold the knife blade and the abrasive is connected to a rod that slides through angle slots above and below the knife's cutting edge. Round diamond-sharpening rods are very difficult to use, as it seems impossible to hold a consistent angle, and therefore more blades are wrecked than sharpened.[4]

Find a motorized knife sharpener! I strongly encourage having a motorized, high-quality diamond-coated, set-angle disc sharpener in your clinic. A 3-stage unit can be found at most department stores for less than $150. Each stage has a slightly different angle for the abrasives. The final stage in these is generally 5° wider, which provides increased durability to the cutting edge. Delegate the sharping to a technician.[4]

Buy lots of knives and keep several sharp knives in your practice vehicle. When purchased in a 6-pack from a packing plant supplier, knives cost approximately 25% less than when purchased singly. Buy high-quality knives. Veterinarians find stiff blades from 6 to 8 inches in length are the best suited for cattle necropsies.[4]

Determining when the edge is sharp

A sharp cutting edge should be smooth and will grab or hold on to a plastic ink pen at a 45° angle when the blade is rested on the pen without sliding down the barrel. If it holds onto the plastic barrel, the cutting edge is sharp.

Finishing the cutting edge and keeping your knife sharp

A ceramic sharpening rod is the best tool found for honing a fine edge on a necropsy knife blade. When using a ceramic rod or metal steel, stroke the blade gently, feeling for defects in the cutting edge as the blade slides down the tool.[4]

Key to keeping your necropsy knife sharp

Beside knives, consider having a boy's 2.25-lb axe, looping shears with extendable handles, utility knife and blades, and a cordless reciprocating saw fitted with a course heavy pruning blade (**Fig. 7**).

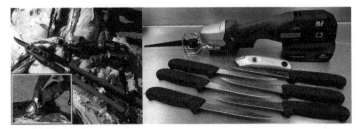

Fig. 7. Necropsy tools.

Do not use your necropsy knife for jobs that will damage its cutting edge. For example, I use a utility (box cutter or carpet) knife for skin incisions to avoid damaging the cutting edge of the necropsy knife on hide, hair, dirt, and/or mud. Additionally, I avoid damaging my necropsy knife blade by not using to cut plastic ID ear tags and cutting rib cartilages, unless the rib cartilages are in very young animals. A lopping shear, axe, or (my new favorite) cordless reciprocating saw saves the cutting edge of the knife.[4]

Feedlot Necropsy Technique That Minimizes Loose Body Parts

Start with the ruminant on its left side

Think about what you are observing and let the lymph nodes be your guide.[4] The structure and function of the organ tissues can be key to linking observations to a meaningful diagnosis.[9,10] Try to connect observations into a unifying diagnosis or production management observation.[4] Be slow to jump to diagnostic conclusion based on your first observations and look at all body systems. The "lift a leg and look" or "peek-a-boo" necropsies generally leave important production management observation undiscovered and minimize the value of the observations that could have contributed to better animal care and management.

Accessing the brain

Important note: rabies should be on the differential of all cattle suffering from CNS disease; therefore, protect yourself and bystanders from contamination. The rabies virus does not survive in dead animals beyond 24 hours when the carcass remains above 70°F.[11]

Cuts through the calvaria with a short-handled axe are made approximately 1.5 cm above the lateral canthus across the forehead and from the lateral canthus dorsally over the pole (**Fig. 8**). Make sure the axe cuts are completely through the cranium. Use the blunt or hammer side of the single-bit axe to strike the cut edge of the cranium along the frontal crest at a 45° angle to break the calvarium away from the brain.

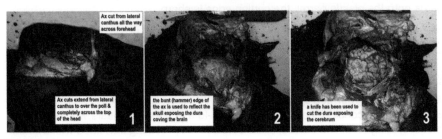

Fig. 8. Brain removal steps.

Removing the brain is a 2-step process. Start by cutting the dura mater across the cerebral falx. The falx is the tough medial division of the dura (see **Fig. 8**). Extend this cut to allow your fingers to slide beneath the cerebrum. Next, cut between the cerebrum and the cerebellum at the level of the pons and lift the cerebrum out of the cranium. The second step requires splitting the dura mater covering the cerebellum dorsally. After the dura covering the cerebellum is cut, slide the tip of your necropsy knife behind the cerebellum into the spinal canal and cut across the spinal cord distal to the obex. Lift out the cerebellum and spinal cord containing the obex.

Opening the hide and reflecting the legs
Keeping the skin incision within a hands breath of the midline will improve the hide value to the rendering company. Therefore, avoid cutting the hide behind the front leg and in front of the back leg. I use a utility knife for all hide incisions. I avoid detaching any organs that are not required to be detached for examination. Detaching organs needlessly creates additional work for rendering company personnel and make a nasty job even harder. Additionally, not detaching organs makes it easier to remove the animal from the necropsy to disposal area with all it parts and is less likely to create a mess at the feedlot.

Using a utility knife, begin cutting along the underside of the jaw continuing over the larynx and down the neck over the trachea. Extend the incision toward the animal's right foreleg axillary space and continue to cut the skin along the ventral thorax across the costochondral junctions, continuing along the abdominal wall toward the right rear inguinal area. The incision across the thorax and abdomen will be a few inches lateral to the midline (see **Fig. 8**).

Reflect the rear leg before attempting to reflect the foreleg. While reflecting the rear leg do not worry about finding the coxofemoral joint. When you cut the heavy muscles (adductor, semimembranosus, pectineus, and sartorius) that hold the coxofemoral joint in place, a sucking sound will be heard as the joint dislocates, exposing the round ligament. Cut the round ligament and examine the joint (**Fig. 9**).

To examine the stifle and hock joints, begin with the rear leg reflected. Skin along the inside of the leg from the stifle joint past the hock joint. Cut along the side of the stifle joint over the femoral trochlea. Next, cut above the patella through its quadriceps attachment down to the femur. Rotate the patella laterally over the condyles. This provides a great view of the stifle joint. To examine the hock joint, cut across the extensor muscles and use the distal bellies of the muscles as a handle for lifting up on the distal tendons as they cross the hock joint. Cut between the tendons and the tibia down to the hock joint. As the joint is approached, you should notice the hock joint capsule. Cut across the joint capsule to expose the joint. Because the tendons are lifting up on the capsule, it usually pops open allowing noncontaminated access for joint fluid collection.

Next, finish skinning the carcass back and reflect the foreleg. Begin by working from the back side and reflect the hide back as you work toward the front leg. As you get to the shoulder, the latissimus dorsi holding the foreleg down will be easily cut. Move to the sternal side of the animal and lift the foreleg, first cutting the pectoral muscles and continue to lift as you cut serratus ventralis muscles. The foreleg should lay over easily with only minor fascia dissection. This approach avoids cutting up the arm pit and lessening the value for the render.

Examining the oral cavity and neck structures
Cut the skin along the side of the cheek, exposing the cheek teeth. A great view of the oral cavity is provided, including an opportunity to examine the tongue, and allows for

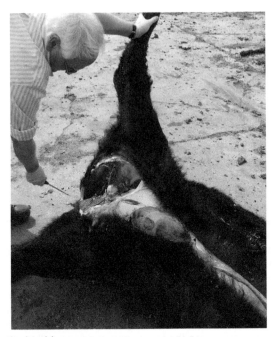

Fig. 9. Reflecting the hind leg.

examining molar eruption (**Fig. 10**). The first molar erupts in cattle at approximately 7 months of age and is in full wear at approximately 12 months.[12] Because almost all feeder cattle are younger than 2 years when arriving at the necropsy area, if age information is useful, the molar eruption is the only clue available, as the incisors do no begin erupting until approximately 20 months of age.

Cut in front of the larynx and dissect the larynx, trachea, and esophagus away from the neck. Open the esophagus, larynx and trachea down to the level of the thoracic

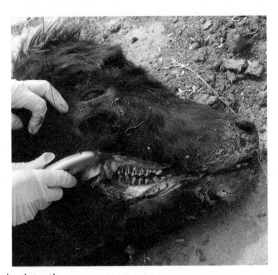

Fig. 10. View of cheek teeth.

inlet for examination. If a "bloat-line" observation is important in the necropsy, separate the esophagus from the trachea down to the thoracic inlet. Later, when the pluck is lifted over the first rib, the esophagus can be withdrawn through the thoracic inlet and its entire length can be examined.

Opening the abdomen and thorax

There are numerous ways to enter the abdomen. I incise the abdominal wall along the greater curvature of the last rib, being careful not to incise the intestine. Once I can get my hand inside the abdomen, I reverse the grip on my necropsy knife so the tip of the handle is forward and, with the knife point outside the abdomen, I slide my hand inside the abdomen with the knife handle leading the cutting edge and incise the abdominal wall as I advance my hand (**Fig. 11**). Continue until the abdominal wall is reflected. Tear the omentum out of the way, exposing the small intestines.

Using a shear, axe, or cordless reciprocating saw, cut across the distal ribs close to the costochondral junctions. The ribs may be separated and manually reflected by breaking the individual ribs back, dislocating the rib from the spine (**Fig. 12**). I leave the first rib intact so I can reflect the pluck over the rib and the rib will hold the pluck off the ground and keep it attached to the carcass, preventing the pluck from falling out as the necropsied animal is removed.

Examining the thoracic cavity

Examine the pericardial sac and fluid. To detach the puck, start by cutting between the thoracic vertebra and aorta. Then dissect the lungs free from the diaphragm. Cut across the aorta, vena cava, esophagus, and mediastinal reflections from the pericardial sac. Continue to free the pluck by cutting the pericardial sac loose from the sternum. Reflect the lungs by grasping the LEFT diaphragmatic lobe and lift the lungs and heart forward over the first rib (**Fig. 13**).

Palpate the lung, and examine the tracheobronchial lymph nodes and airways. The esophagus can be pulled through the thoracic inlet if a potential bloat line is of interest. There are multiple acceptable ways to examine the heart in feeder cattle. I examine the heart's pericardium as I lift the heart. I cut across both ventricles of the heart half way between the apex and the coronary grove. This allow visualization of both heart valves and the left papillary muscles for evidence of necrosis often associated with

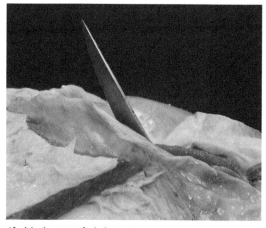

Fig. 11. Holding knife blade out of abdomen.

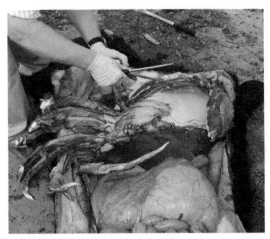

Fig. 12. Exposing the thorax by breaking the ribs back.

Histophilus somni. Open the remaining dorsal ventricles through the aorta and pulmonary artery. These steps are illustrated from left to right in **Fig. 14**.

Examining the abdominal cavity

Fan the small intestines out or spread over the rumen and closely examine the mesenteric lymph nodes (**Fig. 15**). Autolysis can make it pointless to open and examine the entire length of the intestine. Mesenteric lymph nodes usually retain their architecture longer than bowel and examination is useful. Take a look at the ileocecal valve for signs associated with salmonellosis.

When the small intestines are spread over the rumen, it is easy to examine the right kidney and liver. Next, flip the small intestine over the back, exposing the colon, bladder, and left kidney (see **Fig. 15**).

Make a small hole in the rumen behind the anterior pillars. Reach in and find the ruminoreticular fold. Pull the fold to the surface and examine the anterior wall of the ventral blind sac for acidosis lesions or scars.

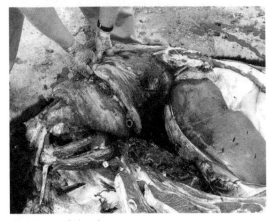

Fig. 13. Pulling the lung out of the thorax.

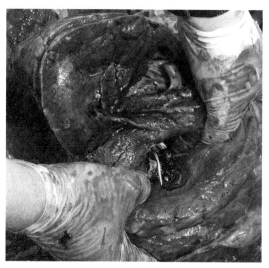

Fig. 14. Heart examination technique.

To reach the spleen, feel under the anteroventral edge of the abomasum next to the diaphragm. Palpate the reticulum for evidence of hardware disease. Open the abomasum to examine the surface for lesions, such as ulcers, parasites, or scarring.

Recording Your Observations

The principal purpose of feedlot necropsies is to gain information that evaluates or can provide clues that can influence production management decisions. Observations, beautifully written, generally get lost in a file drawer and are of little value in analyzing herd-level observations over time. A necropsy observations check-off form improves consistency of observations, especially if necropsies are performed by trained personnel, rather than the veterinarian (**Fig. 16**). A consistent set of digital photographs

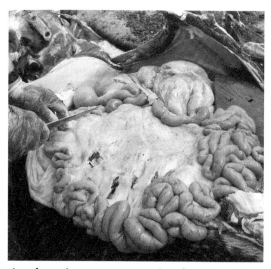

Fig. 15. Small intestines fanned out over rumen, then flip to examine colon.

Date: _____ Yard, Pen/Lot & Animal ID: _____   Samples taken Yes/No

Sex (S-H-B/C) **Breed** (British-Zebu-Exotic-Dairy)   **Weight**: (<4, 4–6, 6–8, 8–10, >10)   **Approx DOF**: _____

Died Where (Receiving, Home, Hosp, Recovery)   **Euthanized** (Y/N)   **Type stress** (Heat-Shipping-Rain-Mud)

L temp: <40 s, 50 s, 60 s, 70 s   **H temp**: <60 s, 70 s, 80 s, 90 s, >100

Pull Dx _____   **Previously Sick** (N-Y: <30 or >30 days)

RxAB: Amp, Baytril, Draxxin, Exc-Exl-Nax, Micotil, Nuflor, OTC, Pen, Sulfa, Zactran, Zuprevo/Mass Med: (Y-N-U)

PHOTO Surface & Opened with ID in pic: **Lung + LN, Heart, Liver, Kidney, Sm. Intestine + Mesenteric LN, Other**

Place an "NE" next to body systems that NOT EXAMINED		
GENERAL CONDITION	**HEART**	**Reproductive**
BCS ( )	Outside infection	Infected
Fresh (F) or Rotten (R)	Inside infection	pregnant (early, mid, late)
	Bloody spots on surface	
SKIN	Enlarged	**JOINTS & BONES**
General hair loss or skin infection		Injury
Sinus injury or infection	**INTESTINE**	Infected
Mammary gland infected	Contents bloody	
	Lymph nodes large	**MUSCLES**
Oral Cavity Lesions (Y/N)	Infection	Neck – bloody
	Peritonitis	Back & side – blood spots
NECK	Obstructed	Hind leg – pale
Bad IV injection		Injection site
Dark blood filled neck	**LIVER**	Muscle injury
	Rotten big yellow spots	
ESOPHAGUS	General yellow color	**SPLEEN**
Ulcers or Erosions	Abscess	Swollen and full of blood
Edema (Parasites)	Migrating Flukes (black streaks)	
	Large Hard Congested (Nutmeg)	**Kidney** (Lf/Rt)
TRACHEA		Abnormal color (Pale/Dark)
Larynx lesion	**GALLBLADDER**	Rough with scars or streaks
Trachea Red or bloody	Enlarged	Bloody spots
Top thick & bloody	Bloody inside surface	Mushy rotten
Froth or fluid in lumen	Bile ducts-Flukes	Infection/Pus
		Bladder – red spots or infected
LUNG	**RUMEN RETICULUM-OMASUM:**	Urine – bloody or flocculent
Fluid around lung	Free Gas	
Lung collapsed	Froth	**BRAIN**
Lung fluid filled	Bloody spots on folds	Dark red and watery
Lung gas/emphysema	Ulcers	Slight pus on the bottom
Lung dark & hard	Traumatic adhesions	Small dark rotten areas
Lung abscesses		Injury
Lung stuck to ribs	**ABOMASUM:**	
Lung lymph node large & angry	Thick folds	**CANCER** … where?
%Affected (<1/3, 1/3–2/3, >2/3)	Ulcers	
Approx Age (<1, 1–3, >3 wks)	Thick with white spots	

Etiology		U = Unknown	Rank Sys & Etiology	Etiology	Rank	Rank Sys & Etiology	Etiology	Rank	Rank Sys & Etiology	Etiology	Rank
C = Circulatory	E = Environ	F = Feed Relate	Gen Body			Skin/SubQ			Musculo-Skeletal		
I = Infectious	M = Metabolic	Ne = Neoplasia	Respiratory			Circ/Hem/Lymph			Gastro-Intestinal		
P = Parasitic	T = Trauma	Tx = Toxic	Urinary			Reproductive			Nervous		

General Comments &/or Diagnosis: _____

Fig. 16. Necropsy observation "check-off" form.

of each necropsy that includes the *animal's identification tag in each photo* can be very valuable when communicating with the removed veterinarian, pathologist, or lawyer. The photos one may take include the surface and opened view of the lung with the tracheobronchial lymph node, heart, kidney, and the small intestine with an associated mesenteric lymph node.

The necropsy form described in a Microsoft Word format, as well as a Microsoft Access necropsy database, that allows necropsy report forms to be easily searched for relationships between cases and production management decisions, can be downloaded from the University of Nebraska–Lincoln, Great Plains Veterinary Educational Center's Internet site (http://GPVEC.UNL.EDU) see "Griffin's Teaching Files" under the "Students Resources" section.[4,13]

Final comment

From time to time, collecting samples and submitting them to your diagnostic laboratory will be appropriate. If the samples are not handled correctly, little additional information can be gained. There are several references available.[12–18] At the very least, put you phone number and the laboratory's phone number next to the addresses, double bag all samples, twist the wires on wire-tie bags, include sufficient absorbent to soak up all transported liquids, and place your paper work in a sealed plastic bag to prevent it from getting wet if should there be a fluid leak.

REFERENCES

1. American Veterinary Medical Association. AVMA guidelines for the euthanasia of animals: 2013 edition. Schaumburg (IL); AVMA; 2013.
2. American Association of Bovine Practitioners. Practical euthanasia of cattle. Auburn (AL): AABP; 2013.
3. National Cattlemen's Beef Association. Beef quality assurance program resources. Centennial (CO): NCBA; 2015.
4. Griffin DD. Griffin's teaching files. Clay Center (NE): University of Nebraska – Lincoln, Great Plains Veterinary Educational Center. Available at: http://gpvec. unl.edu/electives/griffin.asp.
5. Berzinš A, Krukle K, Actinš A, et al. The relative stability of xylazine hydrochloride polymorphous forms. Pharm Dev Technol 2010;15(2):217–22.
6. Federal Food, Drug, and Cosmetic Act (FD&C Act), Section 402(a)(1) or (2), CPG Sec. 675.400 Rendered Animal Feed Ingredients, Revised: 11/13/98. Washington, DC. Available online at: http://www.fda.gov/ICECI/ComplianceManuals/CompliancePolicyGuidanceManual/ucm074717.htm.
7. Meeker DL. Essential rendering, National Renderer's Association. Alexandria (VA): North American Rendering; 2006. p. 3.
8. Gilliam JN, Shearer JK, Woods J, et al. Captive-bolt euthanasia of cattle: determination of optimal-shot placement and evaluation of the Cash Special Euthanizer Kit for euthanasia of cattle. Anim Welf 2012;21(4 Suppl 2):99–102.
9. Jubb KV, Kennedy PC, Palmer N. 3rd edition. Pathology of domestic animals, vol. 3. San Diego (CA): Academic Press; 1985. p. 175–92.
10. Dyce KM, Sack WO, Wensing CJG. Textbook of veterinary anatomy. 3rd edition. Philadelphia: Saunders; 2002. p. 627–760.
11. Rabies: aetiology, epidemiology, diagnosis, prevention, and control references. Paris: OIE, World Organisation for Animal Health; 2014.
12. Cropsey LM. Technical aspects of determining over-age in beef cattle. AABP Proceedings, American Association of Bovine Practitioners, Auburn, AL. 1974. p. 67–71.
13. Griffin DD, Shuck K. Packaging and shipping diagnostic samples. Clay Center (NE): University of Nebraska – Lincoln, Great Plains Veterinary Educational Center; 2011.
14. Griffin DD. Field necropsy of cattle and diagnostic sample submission. Vet Clin North Am Food Anim Pract 2012;28(3):391–405.
15. Safe operating procedures: shipping infectious substances. Lincoln (NE): University of Nebraska-Lincoln, Department of Environmental Health and Safety; 2011.

16. Safe operating procedures: packaging and shipping hazardous materials/ dangerous goods. Lincoln (NE): University of Nebraska-Lincoln, Department of Environmental Health and Safety; 2010.

17. Safe operating procedures: shipping infectious substances with or without dry ice. Lincoln (NE): University of Nebraska-Lincoln, Department of Environmental Health and Safety; 2011.

18. Safe operating procedures: shipping items with dry ice that are not otherwise dangerous goods. Lincoln (NE): University of Nebraska-Lincoln, Department of Environmental Health and Safety; 2011.

Optimizing Feedlot Diagnostic Testing Strategies Using Test Characteristics, Disease Prevalence, and Relative Costs of Misdiagnosis

Miles E. Theurer, DVM, PhD[a], Brad J. White, DVM, MS[b],*,
David G. Renter, DVM, PhD[c]

KEYWORDS

- Epidemiology • Diagnostic tests • Economics • Production medicine

KEY POINTS

- Diagnostic tests are frequently applied in feedlot production medicine and range from clinical observations to advanced physiologic assays.
- Positive and negative predictive values provide the greatest information to veterinarians in terms of how to interpret diagnostic test results; predictive values are determined by prevalence, diagnostic sensitivity, and diagnostic specificity.
- Economic estimates including relative costs and expected frequency of false-positives and false-negatives provide a method for evaluating the overall direct financial effects of implementing different diagnostic strategies.
- The value of retesting initially positive or negative animals changes with prevalence and is varies for different types of diseases.
- Estimates for diagnostic sensitivity, specificity, prevalence, and costs of misdiagnosis are valuable in evaluating appropriate diagnostic strategies.

Disclosure: The authors have nothing to disclose.
[a] Center for Outcomes Research and Education, Kansas State University, Mosier Hall J 118, 1800 Denison Avenue, Manhattan, KS 66506, USA; [b] Department of Clinical Sciences, Kansas State University, Mosier Hall Q 211, 1800 Denison Avenue, Manhattan, KS 66506, USA; [c] Center for Outcomes Research and Education, Kansas State University, Coles Hall 309, 1800 Denison Avenue, Manhattan, KS 66506, USA
* Corresponding author.
E-mail address: bwhite@vet.k-state.edu

Vet Clin Food Anim 31 (2015) 483–493
http://dx.doi.org/10.1016/j.cvfa.2015.05.002
0749-0720/15/$ – see front matter © 2015 Elsevier Inc. All rights reserved.

vetfood.theclinics.com

INTRODUCTION

Diagnostic strategies and interpretation of test results are a common challenge that feedlot practitioners manage on a daily basis. Diagnostic tests are performed to generate information that influences therapeutic, prevention, and disease control decisions. A diagnostic test may be as simple as a combination of clinical signs indicating a disease condition requiring therapy, or more intensive methods of specimen collection for analysis through an external laboratory. Test results may be instantaneous or may require days for a diagnostic laboratory to process and provide the information. Appropriate interpretation of diagnostic results is critical to optimizing therapeutic and preventative programs based on potential test outcomes.

Many diagnostic modalities are available to practitioners, and designing an appropriate diagnostic test strategy involves several basic principles regardless of the specific methods of diagnostic testing. Understanding the best method for interpreting diagnostic tests is critical because the test results may change the clinical decision process and influence animal health actions for the individual or cohort. More information about using and interpreting diagnostic tests is given by McKenna and Dohoo.[1]

This article provides approaches for including information on sensitivity, specificity, prevalence, positive and negative predictive values, and economics that should be considered when implementing a diagnostic testing strategy. Determining an appropriate diagnostic strategy in practice involves understanding the test characteristics, prevalence of disease, and the relative costs of misdiagnosis. **Fig. 1** provides the necessary components to consider in designing and implementing a diagnostic testing strategy for a feedlot cattle population. An opportunity exists to improve diagnostic capabilities in production medicine with the continued advancement of technology, but the evaluation of cost-effectiveness for a specific disease situation is essential for optimizing diagnostic test implementation.

SENSITIVITY AND SPECIFICITY

Diagnostic test accuracy is often reported in terms of diagnostic sensitivity and diagnostic specificity.[1,2] Sensitivity is the proportion of truly diseased animals the test correctly identifies as test positive. Specificity is the proportion of truly healthy animals classified as test-negative. Sensitivity and specificity estimates for diagnostic tests may be calculated by applying the tests to known truly diseased and truly healthy animals and determining the proportion of animals the test correctly identifies. Sensitivity

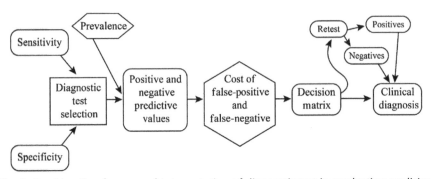

Fig. 1. Consideration for use and interpretation of diagnostic test in production medicine. (*Courtesy of* Mal Hoover, CMI, College of Veterinary Medicine, Kansas State University, Manhattan, KS.)

and specificity estimates also may be determined when no gold standard exists by applying multiple diagnostic tests to the same population of animals or 2 separate populations of animals using more complex analyses,[3] but details and calculation of these methodologies are outside the scope of this article.

Veterinarians typically only know the expected proportion of animals that are diseased and the actual numbers of test positive or negative (apparently diseased and apparently healthy, respectively). **Table 1** lists the potential outcomes when applying a diagnostic test to an animal that could be diseased or healthy. Apparent prevalence is the proportion of the total population that tested positive, and can be determined by applying the test to a population. Animals testing positive are either a true-positive (truly diseased; tested positive) or a false-positive (truly healthy; tested positive). True prevalence is more difficult to determine because the numerator is the sum of the true-positive (truly disease; tested positive) and false-negative (truly diseased; tested negative) animals and the true disease status is rarely known in practice. However, true prevalence influences positive and negative predictive values and thus the practical interpretation of diagnostic test results. The relationship between sensitivity, specificity, and true prevalence determines the relative proportion of correctly and incorrectly classified animals following application of a diagnostic test. Therefore, evaluating all 3 of these variables is critical when designing an optimum diagnostic strategy.

DIAGNOSTIC MODALITIES: EXAMPLES

As examples of diagnostic test strategy selection and implementation, 2 diagnostic modalities with differences in diagnostic accuracies were selected: 1 with a wide range and low diagnostic accuracy (eg, visual observation for bovine respiratory disease [BRD]), and another more accurate diagnostic test (eg, blood test for pregnancy diagnosis). These 2 testing strategies were selected because these examples (BRD and pregnancy diagnosis) are both frequently encountered in feedlot production systems, and the potential diagnostic capabilities are significantly different.

Low and Wide-Ranging Diagnostic Accuracy: Bovine Respiratory Disease Diagnosis

BRD continues to be the most common and economically significant disease affecting feedlot cattle.[4–6] Diagnosis of BRD in field settings is routinely based on visual observations, including depression, anorexia, coughing, nasal discharge, and lack of rumen fill.[7] Observation of clinical signs results in poor and wide-ranging estimates of diagnostic sensitivity and specificity (61.5%–98.9% and 62.8%–94.9%, respectively).[3,8,9] Rectal temperature is a common diagnostic component of BRD diagnosis, but rectal temperature at initial pull for BRD has been shown to have limited accuracy for

Table 1				
Potential outcomes based on diagnostic test results and true disease status				
		True Disease Status		
		Positive	Negative	
Test Result	**Positive**	True-positive	False-positive	Apparent diseased
	Negative	False-negative	True-negative	Apparent healthy
		Truly diseased	Truly healthy	Total population

From these potential outcomes, veterinarians can determine diagnostic sensitivity and specificity estimates, as well as positive and negative predictive value estimates for a given expected prevalence in the population.

predicting whether or not a calf will finish the production cycle.[10] Behavioral activity is also frequently monitored to determine health status in research settings.[11] Even when combining multiple attributes (eg, visual observation of clinical signs, rectal temperature), the sensitivity and specificity of BRD diagnosis are highly variable and low.

On average, 14.4% of all cattle in the feedlot are diagnosed with BRD, but there can be high pen-to-pen variability because 0% to 100% of the animals in a pen may be affected with BRD.[12] Even with a low mean prevalence of BRD, economic consequences related to the severity of BRD still have a significant impact on the feedlot industry. With wide ranges in prevalence estimates for BRD, diagnostic management decisions may need to be changed accordingly in order to reduce the costs of misdiagnosis, appropriately apply therapeutic treatments, and thus optimize economic and clinical outcomes.

Highly Accurate Diagnostic: Bioassay for Pregnancy

Accurate pregnancy diagnosis in heifers can influence appropriate health management decisions in the feedyard.[13,14] Pregnancy diagnosis in feeder heifers can be achieved by rectal palpation, ultrasonography, and blood analysis for bioassay evaluation. The IDEXX bioassay for pregnancy diagnosis has reported sensitivity and specificity estimates of 99.3% and 95.1%, respectively,[15] which is considered a highly accurate test. Pregnancy diagnosis using this assay provides a precise and accurate diagnostic modality for illustrative purposes.

Average pregnancy prevalence in feedlot heifers on arrival has been reported to range from 4.4% to 16.5%.[16–19] However, prevalence can range from 0% to 100% of an individual cohort of cattle. A cohort is a group of animals that were purchased, managed, and marketed similarly, but do not have to be housed in the same pen for the feeding period.[20] Pregnancy can be economically significant even with the low prevalence. Management options for pregnant heifers have been well documented and include administration of an abortifacient to all heifers on arrival to the feedlot, palpation and administration of abortifacient to diagnosed pregnant heifers, or doing nothing and managing potential sequelae as they arise.[13,14,21]

USING SENSITIVITY, SPECIFICITY, AND PREVALENCE TO DETERMINE POSITIVE AND NEGATIVE PREDICTIVE VALUES

Positive predictive value is the proportion of test-positive animals that are truly diseased (true-positive/test positive). Negative predictive value is the proportion of test-negative animals that are truly disease negative (true-negative/test-negative). These predictive values provide direct inferences about the probability of disease given the test result obtained. Prevalence, sensitivity, and specificity all affect predictive values. For most tests, sensitivity and specificity are assumed to not change among different populations, but true prevalence may range widely based on the characteristics of the cattle population.[1] The expected true prevalence values can be established based on the feedlot practitioner's knowledge of historical disease frequency with similar types of cattle. By using expected prevalence, sensitivity and specificity to estimate predictive values, clinicians can be more refined in evaluating diagnostic test results for specific populations by determining the relationships between observed test results and the probability of true disease status.

The importance of interpreting diagnostic tests using positive and negative predictive values can be shown by examining the potential for incorrect classifications based on a changing prevalence (**Fig. 2**). The lower and wider range of sensitivity and specificity estimates resulted in greater chance of misdiagnosis with the BRD example compared

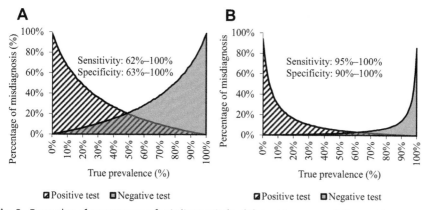

Fig. 2. Examples of percentage of misdiagnosis for (*A*) a wide range of diagnostic accuracy, as with BRD clinical diagnosis; and (*B*) a highly accurate diagnostic test, as with blood test for pregnancy, by true prevalence in the feedlot population.

with the pregnancy test scenario. However, the type of incorrect classification varies based on the disease prevalence. The percentage of incorrect classifications was higher for positive diagnosis (false-positives) in lower-prevalence scenarios, but the expected impact was influenced by the differences in sensitivity and specificity in the two examples. These misclassifications affect overall accuracy, but accuracy, or the overall numbers of misclassifications, is not the only practical consideration because a false-positive or false-negative may have different economic ramifications.

The expected true prevalence influences the predictive values of a test and therefore the chance of false-positive and false-negative results. For the BRD test example, at 10% true prevalence there is a 67% chance of making a misdiagnosis if the test is positive, but only a 3% chance of making a misdiagnosis if the test is negative. As true prevalence increases to 80% for BRD, there is a 5% chance of making a misdiagnosis if the test is positive, but a 50% chance of making a misdiagnosis if the test is negative. This example shows the different interpretations with application of the same test to different populations; in a high-prevalence situation, greater confidence can be placed in positive test results, whereas in the low-prevalence situation positive test results often do not indicate true disease status.

Even when a more accurate test is applied (eg, pregnancy test), the confidence in positive and negative test results varies by expected prevalence. Using the prevalence situations described earlier, with the pregnancy test and true prevalence of 10%, there is a 30% chance of making a misdiagnosis if the test is positive, whereas there is a 0.2% chance of misdiagnosis if the test is negative. As true prevalence increases to 80%, there is a 1% chance of making a misdiagnosis following a positive test, and a 7% chance of misdiagnosis if the test is negative. Thus, the diagnostic characteristics of the test and the prevalence affect the predictive values and the expected frequency of each type of misclassification.

Understanding the primary misclassification (false-negatives or false-positives) in a given test-prevalence situation is critical because this influences diagnostic test interpretation and potential subsequent impacts. Concurrently considering the prevalence, sensitivity, and specificity allows practitioners to determine when to have confidence in positive and negative diagnostic test results. Although distinguishing the individual animals that are misclassified is not possible, an understanding of the relative proportions in the populations enables knowledge-based interpretation of test results. The examples provided in **Fig. 2** show which of the diagnostic test results are most likely to indicate true disease status (true-positive or true-negative) based on multiple prevalence situations for diagnostic tests with 2 different accuracies.

Evaluation of Economic Consequences of Test Misclassifications

Simulation models were developed for the 2 examples of diagnostic testing strategies applied in varied prevalence scenarios to evaluate the total potential cost of misdiagnosis and potential advantage of retesting animals. Simulation models allow the inclusion of distributions for prevalence, diagnostic sensitivity, diagnostic specificity, and economic outcomes in order to evaluate overall impacts of testing scenarios. Test accuracy characteristics for each diagnostic strategy and economic net returns for true-positive, false-positive, false-negative, and true-negative estimates were extracted from published literature evaluating BRD and pregnancy management decisions for feedlot heifers.[14,22] For the purpose of including variability around the estimates of pregnancy bioassay sensitivity and specificity, minimum estimates were established at 95% and 90%, respectively. Baseline economic net return estimates for nonpregnant, pregnant, and aborted heifers were used to develop net-returns estimates for true-negative, false-negative, and true-positive results respectively. Costs for false-positives were fixed at $3.50 per animal relative to nonpregnant heifers because of the expense of administering an abortifacient.

A simulation was performed with 100,000 iterations and a uniform distribution for true prevalence ranging 0% to 100% in order to model impacts of test results over all potential scenarios. Maximum sensitivity and specificity distributions were extended to 100% for the simulation models for BRD and pregnancy diagnosis. For illustrative purposes, results are categorized for each 10% prevalence level (see **Fig. 2**; **Figs. 3** and **4**).

COST OF MISCLASSIFICATIONS (FALSE-POSITIVES AND FALSE-NEGATIVES)

The relative values of misclassifications can influence which diagnostic test characteristic is most critical in different prevalence situations. Theurer and colleagues[22] used a simulation model to show that improving BRD specificity was more valuable than

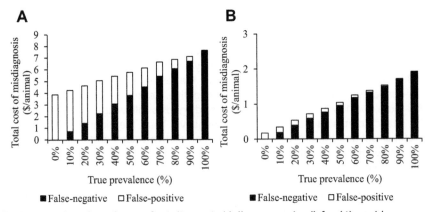

Fig. 3. Examples of total cost of misdiagnosis (dollars per animal) for (A) a wide range of diagnostic accuracy, as with BRD diagnosis; and (B) a highly accurate diagnostic test, as with blood test for pregnancy, by true prevalence in the feedlot population. Note that the scale of the y axis differs between the two charts.

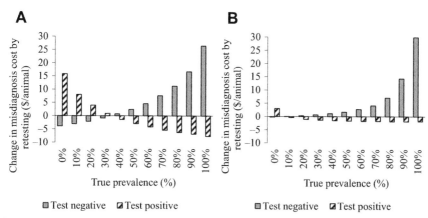

Fig. 4. Examples of the change in misdiagnosis costs (dollars per animal) by retesting positive and negative calves from the initial test for (A) a wide range of diagnostic accuracy, as with BRD; and (B) a highly accurate diagnostic test, as with blood test for pregnancy, by true prevalence in the feedlot population.

sensitivity improvement in populations with both low (<15%) and high (≥15%) apparent prevalence. Wolfger and colleagues[23] evaluated an automated recording system for BRD diagnosis, but the costs of the system were greater than the expected improvement in BRD therapeutic responses. Therefore, the relative costs of misclassification must be compared with the costs of improving diagnostic characteristics in order to optimize the diagnostic testing strategy.

False-negatives incur costs because the animal does not receive therapy appropriate for the true disease condition. The impact of not receiving appropriate therapy is relative to the true-positives that did receive appropriate therapy. In true-positive BRD cases, administering an antibiotic to a calf can reduce mortality risk and improve treatment success.[24] For true-positive pregnancies in feedlot heifers, administering abortifacients results in greater economic returns because of decreased death loss, improved feed/gain ratio, and improved average daily gain.[13,14,21] False-positives incur costs through the application of unnecessary therapies and may result in $15 to $25 per animal (BRD)[25,26] or $3.50 per animal (pregnancy) based on the therapy administered.[14]

The costs of misdiagnosis are relative to the value of accurate identification of the true disease status. For truly diseased animals, compare the relative costs of a false-negative with a true-positive, and for truly healthy animals compare the costs of a false-positive with the economic value of a true-negative. For both BRD and pregnancy diagnosis examples, false-negative animals had lower net returns than false-positive animals. The lower net return in false-negative animals is caused by the potential benefit of a therapeutic treatment being greater than the costs of treating an animal that is truly healthy. However, for BRD, antibiotics are not 100% effective in preventing death. The absolute risk reduction for BRD mortality ranges from 2.5% to 44%, with the median value being 17%.[22,24] The low efficacy of antibiotics for BRD mortality risk means that, for every 6 animals treated therapeutically for BRD, 1 death is prevented (using the median estimate of the absolute risk reduction).[24] The distribution of antibiotic efficacy estimates was included in our simulations for determining the economic net returns in true-positive animals for BRD. For pregnancy in feedlot heifers, abortifacients are effective for inducing labor and causing an abortion; abortifacient efficacy is reported to be 95%.[27] Because of the higher efficacy of the pregnancy treatment compared with BRD antibiotic treatment, the relative costs of false-negative and true-positive test results were greater for pregnancy misdiagnosis compared with BRD misdiagnosis.

Fig. 3 shows the total costs of misdiagnosis for different levels of prevalence for BRD and pregnancy scenarios respectively. When BRD prevalence is low, the total cost of misdiagnosis is primarily caused by false-positives, as shown in **Fig. 3**A. For pregnancy diagnosis, **Fig. 3**B shows that costs for false-negatives comprise most of the total costs of misdiagnosis when prevalence is greater than 10%. The total cost of misdiagnosis increases for both BRD and pregnancy scenarios as the true prevalence increases. This increase in total costs of misdiagnosis is caused by false-negatives costing more than false-positives, and the frequency of false-negatives increases with increasing prevalence when sensitivity is not perfect (<100%).

The cost of false-positives differs based on the specific disease scenario. For example, false-positives for bovine diarrhea virus (BVD) have greater potential economic consequences than false-positives for BRD. With suggested restrictions in marketing BVD-positive animals,[28,29] a calf diagnosed as BVD positive potentially loses all economic value. Both the costs and probabilities of false-positive and false-negative results should be taken into account in determining an optimal diagnostic testing strategy.

DECISION MATRIX FOR OPTIMIZING DIAGNOSTIC STRATEGIES

The decision matrix in this instance is the process of considering modifications to a diagnostic testing strategy based on changes to total misdiagnosis costs through retesting the animals categorized as positive or negative based on the initial test. The process is used to determine whether it is economically feasible to consider retesting individuals to improve diagnostic certainty, or to proceed in applying health interventions based only on the results from the initial test. This decision requires information on the accuracy of the diagnostic test used for the initial test, the relative costs of initial false-positive and false-negative results compared with those correctly classified, the number of animals that will initially be tested, the accuracy of the diagnostic test used for retesting, and costs of retesting. For illustrative purposes with our examples, sensitivity and specificity estimates of the new, independent diagnostic test used for retesting was assumed to have the same values as the original test.

RETEST THE POSITIVE OR NEGATIVE ANIMALS FROM THE INITIAL TEST

Retesting positive or negative animals may reduce the costs of misdiagnosis, but an economic analysis is necessary to determine the potential value of this change. To calculate the economic impact of retesting, it is necessary to estimate the change in the total cost of misdiagnosis that is achieved by retesting positive or negative animals from the initial test, the number of animals that would be retested, and the diagnostic accuracy of the retest used.

The change in total costs of misdiagnosis are not as intuitive to interpret as the initial total cost of misdiagnosis, because there are some situations in which retesting animals results in increased total costs of misdiagnosis because of a greater frequency of diagnostic errors. In a high-prevalence situation, retesting animals that initially tested positive results in economic loss by increasing the total costs of misdiagnosis. This increased cost of misdiagnosis is primarily caused by imperfect diagnostic sensitivity of the second test and some diseased animals initially being classified as positive that are now be classified as false-negative based on the retest. Although there would be fewer false-positive animals following retesting of initially positive animals, the overall negative economic returns result from the increased number of false-negative animals and the cost of false-negatives exceeding the benefits of reducing false-positives. A similar scenario arises when retesting negative animals in a low-prevalence situation that also results in a greater total cost of misclassification. Retesting animals with less than a perfect test (<100% sensitivity and specificity) does not eliminate diagnostic errors, so when considering the usefulness of retesting it is critical to determine how retesting changes the numbers of misclassifications and what costs are associated with each type of misdiagnosis.

Fig. 4 shows the changes in costs of misdiagnosis for the BRD and gives examples of pregnancy diagnosis for different prevalence situations. Considering the change in misdiagnosis costs in terms of dollars per animal is important in determining how much the clinician can afford to pay for retesting individual animals. This analysis is performed by evaluating the change in costs of misdiagnosis divided by frequency of calves that initially tested positive or negative in the population. Retesting positive or negative animals may decrease the costs of misdiagnosis; however, the economic viability of this strategy is influence by the expected proportion of misdiagnosis, cost of the secondary test, and relative cost of misdiagnosis compared with accurate diagnosis.

For a 10% BRD prevalence, it would be economically beneficial to retest the positive animals as long as the diagnostic test costs less than $8 per animal. Using an increased rectal temperature as a follow-up diagnostic test for animals deemed BRD positive in the pen is inexpensive and this method is commonly used to determine whether the animal should receive an antibiotic for treatment of BRD. However, Fig. 4A shows that, when true prevalence exceeds 40%, it may be more economically beneficial to avoid retesting animals initially testing positive, and to reevaluate the animals initially considered healthy (initial test-negatives). When prevalence is 80%, it is economically beneficial to retest negative animals if the second diagnostic test costs less than $11. Values like these are useful to determine how much it may be reasonable to pay for retesting and still result in an economic benefit. There are multiple prevalence values for which it may not be appropriate to retest animals, because of the low frequency and costs of initial misdiagnosis.

With the pregnancy testing scenario, there is less economic incentive to retest positive or negative animals. There is a wide range of true-prevalence values for which it is not economically beneficial to retest positive or negative animals because of the negligible change in the total cost of misdiagnosis and the number of animals that would need to be retested to change the economic outcome. The difference between the BRD and pregnancy diagnosis scenarios with respect to the change in costs of misdiagnosis is primarily driven by the better and less variable sensitivity and specificity estimates for the pregnancy test compared with BRD diagnosis. Thus, having a more accurate initial diagnostic test results in less potential for improving misdiagnosis and economic benefits with follow-up testing.

There are inherent advantages and disadvantages of using retesting to improve overall diagnostic sensitivity or specificity, and the corresponding economic impacts of misdiagnosis, and these effects vary with prevalence. However, there is rarely, if ever, a diagnostic test that provides the correct answer for both positive and negative results (100% sensitivity and specificity estimates). Retesting the positive animals or the negative animals from the initial test may be reasonable if the practitioner is concerned with the impacts of false-positive or false-negative results, respectively (see Fig. 2). However the economic consequences of retesting can vary greatly based on the test characteristics and the prevalence, as shown in Fig. 4.

SUMMARY

Optimizing diagnostic strategies for feedlot populations requires knowledge of the diagnostic test characteristics, the expected prevalence for the population, and the potential costs or impacts of incorrect diagnoses. Incorporating information on economic costs and benefits of different diagnostic strategies provides a mechanism to comprehensively evaluate diagnostic scenarios. Costs of misdiagnosis should be considered in relation to benefits realized by correctly classifying individuals (ie, compared with those that receive the appropriate treatment or health intervention) to improve the clinical and economic outcomes. There also may be instances in which animal welfare and public perception considerations may need to be taken into account as well when determining the decision process to arrive at the clinical diagnosis. The potential benefits of decisions based on test results can vary based on test accuracy as well as on the disease prevalence in the population.

A spreadsheet with input cells for sensitivity, specificity, prevalence, and estimated costs of misdiagnosis can be created in order to evaluate diagnostic strategies, including estimating the potential value of retesting animals. The exact values for test accuracy, prevalence, and costs of misdiagnosis are not essential, but reasonable estimates can be considered in order to make sound clinical and economic decisions. The example data provided in the text and figures here are not meant to show exact costs of misdiagnosis or the amount to spend for retesting, but are used as examples of the proposed principles and methods. Using these concepts in practice could enhance the application of diagnostic strategies to optimize clinical and economic outcomes.

ACKNOWLEDGMENTS

The authors acknowledge Mal Hoover at Kansas State University for helping to prepare **Fig. 1** for publication.

REFERENCES

1. McKenna SL, Dohoo IR. Using and interpreting diagnostic tests. Vet Clin North Am Food Anim Pract 2006;22(1):195–205.
2. Dohoo I, Martin W, Stryhm H. Veterinary epidemiologic research. Charlottetown (Canada): AVC Inc; 2009.
3. White BJ, Renter DG. Bayesian estimation of the performance of using clinical observations and harvest lung lesions for diagnosing bovine respiratory disease in post-weaned beef calves. J Vet Diagn Invest 2009;21(4):446–53.
4. Galyean ML, Perino LJ, Duff GC. Interaction of cattle health/immunity and nutrition. J Anim Sci 1999;77(5):1120–34.
5. Lechtenberg K, Daniels C, Royer G, et al. Field efficacy study of gamithromycin for the control of bovine respiratory disease in cattle at high risk of developing the disease. Int J Appl Res Vet Med 2011;9(2):184–92.
6. Griffin D. Economic impact associated with respiratory disease in beef cattle. Vet Clin North Am Food Anim Pract 1997;13(3):367–77.
7. Smith RA, Stokka GL, Radostits O, et al. Health and production management in beef feedlots. In: Radostits O, editor. Herd health: food animal production medicine. 3rd edition. Philadelphia: WB Saunders Company; 2001. p. 592–5.
8. Amrine DE, White BJ, Larson R, et al. Precision and accuracy of clinical illness scores, compared with pulmonary consolidation scores, in Holstein calves with experimentally induced *Mycoplasma bovis* pneumonia. Am J Vet Res 2013; 74(2):310–5.

9. Leruste H, Brscic M, Heutinck LF, et al. The relationship between clinical signs of respiratory system disorders and lung lesions at slaughter in veal calves. Prev Vet Med 2012;105(1–2):93–100.

10. Theurer ME, White BJ, Larson RL, et al. Relationship between rectal temperature at first treatment for bovine respiratory disease complex in feedlot calves and the probability of not finishing the production cycle. J Am Vet Med Assoc 2014;245(11):1279–85.

11. Theurer ME, Amrine DE, White BJ. Remote noninvasive assessment of pain and health status in cattle. Vet Clin North Am Food Anim Pract 2013;29(1):59–74.

12. US Department of Agriculture, Animal and Plant Health Inspection Service. Treatment of respiratory disease in U.S. feedlots. 2001.

13. Rademacher RD, Warr BN, Booker CW. Management of pregnant heifers in the feedlot. Vet Clin North Am Food Anim Pract 2015;31(2):209–28.

14. Buhman MJ, Hungerford LL, Smith DR. An economic risk assessment of the management of pregnant feedlot heifers in the USA. Prev Vet Med 2003;59(4):207–22.

15. IDEXX Laboratories I. IDEXX bovine pregnancy test. Available at: https://www.idexx.com/pdf/en_us/livestock-poultry/lpd-bovine-pregnancy-test-sell-sheet.pdf. Accessed March 9, 2015.

16. Edwards AJ, Laudert SB. Economic evaluation of the use of feedlot abortifacients. Bov Pract 1984;19:148–50.

17. Laudert SB. Incidence of pregnancy in feedlot heifers at slaughter. Paper presented at: Cattlemen's Day. Manhattan (KS), March 1988.

18. Bennett BW, Clayton RP, Cravens RL, et al. Slaughter weight loss attributable to pregnancy in feedlot heifers. Mod Vet Pract 1984;65(9):677–9.

19. US Department of Agriculture. Part I: management practices on US feedlots with capacity of 1,000 or more head. Fort Collins (CO): National Animal Health Monitoring System; 2013.

20. Babcock AH, Renter DG, White BJ, et al. Temporal distributions of respiratory disease events within cohorts of feedlot cattle and associations with cattle health and performance indices. Prev Vet Med 2010;97(3–4):198–219.

21. Jim GK, Ribble CS, Guichon PT, et al. The relative economics of feeding open, aborted, pregnant feedlot heifers. Can Vet J 1991;32(10):613–7.

22. Theurer ME, White BJ, Larson RL, et al. A stochastic model to determine the economic value of changing diagnostic test characteristics for identification of cattle for treatment of bovine respiratory disease. J Anim Sci 2015;93(3):1398–410.

23. Wolfger B, Manns BJ, Barkema HW, et al. Evaluating the cost implications of a radio frequency identification feeding system for early detection of bovine respiratory disease in feedlot cattle. Prev Vet Med 2015;118(4):285–92.

24. DeDonder KD, Apley MD. A review of the expected effects of antimicrobials in bovine respiratory disease treatment and control using outcomes from published randomized clinical trials with negative controls. Vet Clin North Am Food Anim Pract 2015;31(1):97–111.

25. US Department of Agriculture. Part III: health management and biosecurity in U.S. feedlots, 1999. Fort Collins (CO): National Animal Health Monitoring System; 2000. #N336.1200.

26. US Department of Agriculture. Types and costs of respiratory disease treatments in U.S. feedlots. 2013.

27. Barth AD, Adams WM, Manns JG, et al. Induction of abortion in feedlot heifers with a combination of cloprostenol and dexamethasone. Can Vet J 1981;22(3):62–4.

28. Academy of Veterinary Consultants. BVD position statement. 2006.

29. American Association of Bovine Practitioners. AABP position statement on disclosure of BVD PI animals. 2007.

Using Feedlot Operational Data to Make Valid Conclusions for Improving Health Management

Miles E. Theurer, DVM, PhD[a], David G. Renter, DVM, PhD[b],*, Brad J. White, DVM, MS[c]

KEYWORDS

- Epidemiology • Feedlot • Data • Distribution

KEY POINTS

- Operational data can be useful, because often they are from the same production system(s) in which the conclusions would be applied; however, some limitations need to be considered to make appropriate conclusions.
- Data need to be assessed for quality and analyzed appropriately before being used for decision making.
- Data errors that are differential, with respect to the populations of animals to be compared, can lead to biased conclusions regarding outcomes and health management factors.
- There is a high potential for confounding in operational data; a practical solution is to partition (ie, stratify) data into comparable population subsets.
- Knowledge of the underlying distribution of health outcome data and the distribution of health events over time can enable more comprehensive evaluations and appropriate conclusions.

INTRODUCTION

Feedlot practitioners often have access to data collected directly from their client's feedlot operations. These operational data can be useful for monitoring the health and performance of feedlot cattle populations. In addition, these data may be used to assess associations between health outcomes and potentially important cattle

The authors have nothing to disclose.
[a] Center for Outcomes Research and Education, Kansas State University, Mosier Hall J 118, 1800 Denison Avenue, Manhattan, KS 66506, USA; [b] Center for Outcomes Research and Education, Kansas State University, Coles Hall 309, 1800 Denison Avenue, Manhattan, KS 66506, USA; [c] Department of Clinical Sciences, Kansas State University, Mosier Hall Q 211, 1800 Denison Avenue, Manhattan, KS 66506, USA
* Corresponding author.
E-mail address: drenter@vet.k-state.edu

Vet Clin Food Anim 31 (2015) 495–508
http://dx.doi.org/10.1016/j.cvfa.2015.05.004
0749-0720/15/$ – see front matter © 2015 Elsevier Inc. All rights reserved.

population or management factors (ie, risk factors) that influence these outcomes. A common question may be: is this factor associated with a health outcome of interest? The potential risk factor (or protective factor) may include items like individual animal or group (ie, lot, pen) characteristics, health management procedures or programs, treatment protocols, or environmental factors. Outcomes frequently monitored include health outcomes of morbidity, mortality, first treatment success, and case fatality risks, and also performance outcomes such as average daily gain, feed to gain conversion, and carcass characteristics. Data can be evaluated to determine if there are associations with the risk factor and outcome of interest and to develop management protocols tailored to specific situations. By quantifying potential associations, practitioners may identify areas to focus resources for improving feedlot cattle health.

Operational data can be relevant and useful resources, because they can be directly representative of the cattle populations and management systems with which a practitioner works on a daily basis. If data are used to drive health management decisions, these decisions could be applied to similar cattle in similar environments and management systems; thus, conclusions from the data could be directly applicable. Although some experimental research trials also may be relevant, often, these types of studies tend to minimize variation in the cattle population, environment, and management to more efficiently evaluate a specific treatment effect(s). When there are fundamental differences in production settings or animal populations between experimental studies and commercial animal management systems, it may be difficult to assess or quantify how well experimental results apply to commercial settings.

Another advantage of using operational data is that large quantities of data may be already collected and available to be used. However, the use of operational data has some limitations, because they are observational in nature: the health outcomes, and factors potentially associated with these outcomes, were observed and not derived within the same structured framework as they would be in a randomized clinical trial. The distribution of cattle characteristics or management factors are not randomly allocated in a commercial cattle population but are often caused by conscious management decisions that can be directly or indirectly related to potential health outcomes. Therefore, risk factors or protective factors that are observed in operational data may not be causally related to the health outcome of interest and may even be spurious findings resulting from confounding effects in the data. Confounding can occur if there is an extraneous factor(s) (one not included in the analysis) that is associated with both the outcome and risk factor of interest. Multiple population factors need to be carefully considered before accurate conclusions can be made from operational data.

There are many operational data resources potentially available for feedlot practitioners; however, accurate and useful information is derived from these data only when the advantages and limitations of the data and the analysis process are fully understood. The objective of this review is to outline some uses, advantages, and limitations of using operational data to assess health outcomes of feedlot cattle and make related health management conclusions. Without appropriate knowledge of key principles and methods of using operational data, wrong conclusions may be made, and corresponding management changes may not have the desired effect on the outcome(s) of interest.[1] The progressive feedlot veterinarian may use this information to make more informed recommendations as more data become available in the information age.

QUANTITY AND QUALITY OF OPERATIONAL DATA

Big data is a term that is used to describe large volumes of data collected and used to make decisions.[2] Record systems are used to capture data in many areas, from the business world to veterinary medicine. The use of big data sets can be beneficial to monitor outcomes or determine associations between outcomes of interest and a wide variety of potential risk factors. The inferences from large feedlot operational data sets may be beneficial in more accurately assessing or predicting health and performance parameters for cattle to develop more appropriate health and economic risk management.

Data precision influences the ability to accurately evaluate outcomes and potential associations with risk factors. If nondifferential error (or random error) in the data is substantial, the effect of interest would have to be larger to recognize the effect. For example, if animal body weights were measured on a scale with 22.7-kg (50-lb) increments, there would be low data precision, or substantial nondifferential error; this would be nondifferential error if occurring similarly for all cattle groups. In this case, recognizing a potential difference in body weights among groups would be difficult unless the true difference, or magnitude of effect, was large. The inaccuracies of the weight measurements results in a significant amount of noise, or variability, in the data, making it more difficult to detect a difference, even if one truly exists.

Current technology enables the ability to easily capture volumes of data on multiple factors, yet, the quality of data needs to be considered before it can be translated into useful information. The use of computerized records, in theory, should reduce data errors and enable data formatting that is more readily used for analysis and interpretation. Examples in human medicine have shown how computerized data entry forms may be used to reduce medication errors by not having to interpret handwriting, automating dosage calculations, and improving identification of the prescribing physician.[3] However, 1 study of handheld computers in human medicine indicated that there were 675 errors per 10,000 entry fields, which is greater than the acceptable rate of 10 errors per 10,000 fields using paper-based double data entry methods.[4,5] Computerized health records have become more available in veterinary medicine, yet, data errors are still a potential concern. These types of errors include typographic errors, miscoding, data merged into the wrong field(s), and other factors that may lead to misinformation even before the data are evaluated for analysis and conclusions.[6-8] Data entry errors can have substantial effects on the outcome(s) measures and can change the magnitude and direction of associations between a risk factor and the outcome of interest.[6,9] Although computerized methods are used to capture and store feedlot data, compiling the data into formats for appropriately assessing health outcomes can still require additional effort.

Each data set should be evaluated to make sure the data are of adequate quality before conclusions are made. One way to detect data errors is to check the data set for obscure values by generating descriptive statistics. This check can be performed by simply determining minimum and maximum values for the variable to identify observations that are outside the expected range or not biologically plausible. In addition, graphically showing the data using histograms can be useful for to identifying potential errors. If data errors are identified and correct information is not able to be determined, consideration of removal of the observations from the data set may be necessary before any analyses. If data errors occur uniformly throughout the data set, then, errors may be nondifferential, because they occurred for all cattle groups in the data set. Identification and correction of data errors can improve data quality, but the underlying cause of the errors should be evaluated to improve the system for future use.

A common misconception with evaluating large data sets is that the very large numbers of records can overcome the potential impact of data errors. However, data errors should be minimized, because the lack of precision can be profound and the effects on conclusions may not be easily determined. Lack of precision can lead to an inability to detect important effects in production systems data, and errors that lead to confounding or bias (differential error, as described later) cannot be overcome simply by the increasing the volume of data. There are no statistical analyses that can be performed to turn poor data into high-quality data. Practitioners should consider carefully the quality of the available operational data, including how and why data were collected, to assess whether the data may be useful for their purposes.

MAKING APPROPRIATE CONCLUSIONS: POTENTIAL FOR DIFFERENTIAL ERRORS IN OPERATIONAL DATA

Feedlot practitioners may often want to use operational data to compare health outcomes among different cattle populations, including those that were managed differently or were fed during different periods or at different sites. Often, these comparisons lead to causal-type conclusions; if outcomes differ among populations, the assumption may be that the evaluated factor(s) caused the observed differences in outcomes. These types of conclusions should be avoided, or at least made with extreme caution, because of the inherent limitations with operational data. One of the concerns is the potential for differential error or bias. Differential error is a systematic error that may result in an incorrect estimate of the association between a factor and outcome of interest.[10] The term is differential because the errors occur at a different frequency between the groups that are being compared (information bias) or because the population being studied differs substantially from the population in which conclusions are meant to be applied (selection bias).[10] Considering the examples of data errors described earlier, if these errors occurred at a different frequency among different cattle populations being compared, it could be a form of information bias that leads to inappropriate conclusions and even changes in health management protocols that do not have the desired impact(s).

As an example, if a practitioner wanted to compare morbidity risk in light-weight steers in a feedlot with morbidity risk in light-weight steers on a wheat pasture, both the frequency and accuracy of morbidity (outcome) monitoring would need to be the same for both groups. Otherwise, differential errors, and thus biased conclusions, could occur. As a simple example, if the feedlot steers were monitored every day for signs of morbidity, there would be more opportunities for each calf to be correctly (or incorrectly) diagnosed, because pen riders may detect subtle change in cattle behavior, resulting in increased morbidity diagnoses.[11] In contrast, if the wheat pasture calves were monitored only once a week for morbidity, then, the morbidity frequency measures, and potentially the accuracy of those measures, would be different between groups, and thus, direct comparisons should not be made.

The potential for differential error also can be high when comparing cattle populations over time using historical data. Cattle characteristics or health management protocols may change over time, which could lead to confounding (described later). In addition, differential error could occur if the accuracy of measured health outcomes or risk factors is different in different periods. For example, feedlot personnel may receive enhanced training in recognizing disease or capturing data on factors that affect disease, which could change the accuracy of outcome or risk factors measurements, respectively. Or the personnel responsible for identifying disease may have changed over the period examined. In this case, comparisons made between periods may be biased, because of errors in outcome or because risk factor measurements have changed over time (ie, risk factors are differential with respect to time). Improvements in health diagnostics over time often make historical comparisons difficult, if not impossible.

The examples of differential errors described earlier would be classified as information bias. However, selection bias can also occur if the population being evaluated differs substantially from the population in which conclusions are meant to be applied. For example, if data from harvested cattle are used to measure the frequency of disease outcomes or the potential association with risk factors, conclusions from those data should be applied only to cattle that are harvested and not to a broader cattle population. With some diseases, it may be likely that harvested cattle differ significantly from the overall cattle population in the feedlot (which also includes cattle that will be culled or will die before harvest). Therefore, the results from harvest audits, although useful, should not be assumed to representative all feeder cattle.

In the presence of differential error, results from operational data sets may be misleading, and thus, conclusions and inferences can be incorrect. Increasing the number of observations (volume of data) does not overcome the pitfalls of differential errors. Evaluating and using operational data sets requires knowledge of biology and the production system, as well as a high level of data scrutiny, to come to appropriate conclusions. Before comparing outcomes among different populations, a practitioner needs to consider some of the potential impacts of differential errors. If the practitioner believes that there is enough potential differential error to lead to biased conclusions, then, conclusions from the data should not be made.

MAKING APPROPRIATE COMPARISONS: IDENTIFYING AND CONTROLLING CONFOUNDING

As indicated earlier, a feedlot practitioner may want to use operational data to compare health outcomes of interest among different cattle populations to assess the potential impacts of specific factors (ie, risk factors). Appropriate comparisons, and thus valid conclusions, can be made only if confounding factors are identified and their effects are controlled. If there is an extraneous factor (confounder) that is significantly associated with both the outcome(s) and risk factor(s) of interest, then, there is the significant potential for confounding.[10] Confounding effects can be common in operational data and can profoundly distort the effect of interest.

As an example of this concept, imagine evaluating the impact of antimicrobial administration at arrival (metaphylaxis) by comparing morbidity risks (outcome) in cattle groups that received metaphylaxis with those that did not receive metaphylaxis (risk factor). In experimental studies, metaphylaxis has been shown to reduce morbidity risk by 53% and reduce mortality risk by 27% compared with cattle that did not receive metaphylaxis.[12] However, in feedlot operational data, the use of metaphylaxis is not randomly applied to different groups of cattle as it would be in an experiment. In operational data, the groups of cattle that did and did not receive metaphylaxis were likely different based on several factors (potential confounders) that are also associated with morbidity risk (outcome). Thus, the factors that are associated with the decision for metaphylaxis administration (ie, the factors used to determine high-risk vs low-risk designation) may completely confound the measure of the impact of metaphylaxis on the outcome (morbidity). We cannot accurately estimate the impact of metaphylaxis (factor of interest) in groups that differ with respect to other (confounding) factors that are also inherently associated with morbidity (outcome of interest). Although this example is extreme, it shows the concept of confounding, which can have profound impacts on conclusions made using operational data.

To reduce the potential impact of confounding, one needs to ask: are the populations that I wish to compare equivalent other than the risk factor(s) of interest? Am I comparing apples with apples? For example, **Fig. 1**A shows aggregated mortality

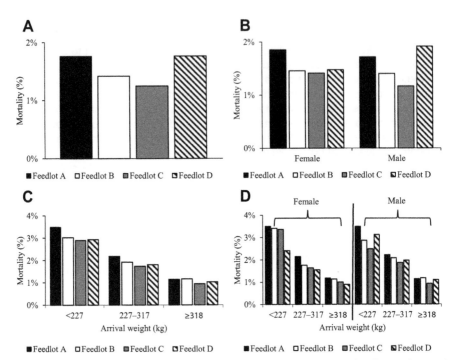

Fig. 1. Average mortality risk by feedlot (*A*), feedlot and sex (*B*), feedlot and arrival weight (*C*), and feedlot, sex, and arrival weight (*D*) for 19,906 lots of cattle from 4 commercial feedlots.

data from multiple feedlots. With data like these, it may be tempting to conclude that some feedlots (factor of interest) are better or worse at health management, because mortality (outcome of interest) seems to differ. However, we know that the type of cattle is not always the same in different feedlots and that the type of cattle can affect mortality; therefore, the potential for confounding exists when comparing mortality among feedlots. Known potential confounders with respect to health outcomes in feedlot operational data may include animal age (calf vs yearling) or arrival weight, sex or castration status, previous management history (preconditioning or vaccination status), and even season of placement.[13] So, if the goal is to appropriately compare mortality risks among feedlots (eg, see **Fig. 1**A), there is a need to make sure that there are no extraneous factors or confounders that (1) differ among feedlots and (2) are associated with the outcome of interest (mortality).

If there are known potential confounding factors, then, this issue must be addressed or valid comparisons cannot be made. There are multiple potential ways to control for confounding factors, but restricting or partitioning the data is likely the most practical approach when using feedlot operational data. A practitioner may restrict comparisons of health outcomes to only a subset of the total population (eg, compare only light-weight steers arriving in the month of October). By restricting the analysis to a specific population, the potential for confounding effects of extraneous factors (in this case, weight, sex, and season) can be reduced and more appropriate comparisons and conclusions may be possible. However, limiting the comparisons to only a subset of the population also limits the scope of the potential conclusions (ie, it does not provide information on the whole cattle population). Thus, if the analysis evaluates only light-weight steers arriving in the month of October, then, the inferences from the results are applicable only to light-weight steers arriving in the month of October.

Another practical way to control for potential confounding in operational data is to partition or stratify the data in to data subsets for appropriate comparisons. Partitioning the data into multiple subsets or strata based on known potential confounders can enable more appropriate and comprehensive comparisons. For example, **Fig. 1**B–D was created by partitioning the aggregated feedlot mortality data (see **Fig. 1**A) so comparisons could be made within subsets of the population based on sex and arrival weight. **Fig. 1**C shows that there is a large apparent difference in mortality risk in different arrival weight categories; across all feedlots, the lighter-weight calves had a greater mortality risk compared with heavier cattle. Therefore, if the distribution of arrival weights differs among feedlots, comparing mortality risks among feedlots, as in **Fig. 1**A, without partitioning the data by arrival weight could result in inappropriate conclusions as a result of confounding effects of arrival weight. **Fig. 1**D further partitions the same data and shows the mortality risk for each feedlot by arrival weight category and sex. There are minimal apparent differences in mortality risk among feedlots when comparing within subsets of the population categorized by arrival weight and sex (see **Fig. 1**D), which may be different from the potential conclusion based on the initial comparison of feedlots with aggregated data (see **Fig. 1**A). Although other factors also may need to be considered, this partitioning or stratifying process reduces the potential confounding effects that could occur when comparing feedlots with cattle populations that may differ with respect to sex and arrival weight (known potential confounders).

A practitioner may want to use operational data to evaluate the potential effects of single factor on an outcome of interest. However, to evaluate these associations appropriately, one may need to control for known potential confounders that can otherwise distort the results from a single risk factor analysis. In our example, there were potentially real differences in the number of mortalities that occur at each of the 4 different feedlots (see **Fig. 1**A). However, there is a need to avoid concluding that feedlots differ in their health management ability, especially when there are known potential confounders such as arrival weight and sex that differ among the feedlots and are associated with the outcome (mortality). Feedlots A and D may have had apparently greater mortality risks (see **Fig. 1**A) simply because the cattle population in those feedlots comprised a higher proportion of lighter-weight calves. Without controlling for potential confounding effects, inappropriate conclusions may be made, which result in changes in health management protocols that may have limited or adverse effects on improving the health outcome(s) of interest.

DISTRIBUTIONS OF POPULATION HEALTH OUTCOMES

It is often tempting to evaluate health outcomes or health management decisions in a feedlot population by using summary statistics (eg, using averages). However, often, the distribution of health outcomes in a feedlot population is not well described using an average (mean) or other measures of central tendency such as a median. This point can be shown by visualizing the frequency distribution of outcomes in a histogram (eg, those in **Fig. 2**), which show the full distribution of observed outcomes. Knowledge of the underlying frequency distributions for each outcome evaluated may need to be understood to make appropriate conclusions. The mean, median, and distribution for morbidity, mortality, first treatment success, and case fatality outcomes in a subset of cattle lots from 23 commercial feedlots over a 6-year period with a minimum of 1 morbidity diagnosis in each lot are shown in **Fig. 2**. These graphs show

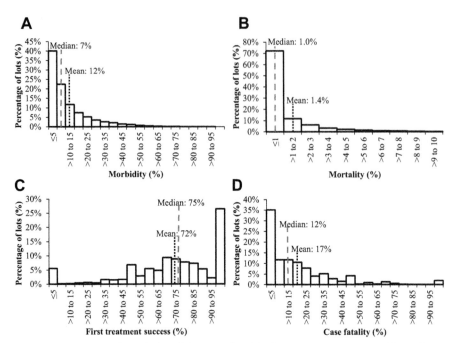

Fig. 2. Distributions of morbidity (*A*), mortality (*B*), first treatment success (*C*), and case fatality (*D*) risks for 33,309 cattle lots representing a subset of the population from 23 commercial feedlots over a 6-year period with a minimum of 1 morbidity diagnosis. Mean (*black dotted line*) and median (*gray dashed line*) values for each distribution shown. Notice the scale of the y-axis differs between the charts.

relationships between the outcome distributions and measures of central tendency (eg, mean and median) in feedlot data and enable an understanding of why the full distribution is often more informative and useful for assessing health outcomes.

Morbidity and mortality risks are often right skewed or positively skewed (eg, see **Fig. 2**A, B, respectively). Skewed distributions occur when there are relatively infrequent observations with very high or low values relative to most observations for the outcome. In this case, the right-skewed distributions occur because a few lots have relatively high morbidity and mortality, and this leads to a long tail in the distributions toward the right. Right-skewed distributions occur more frequently than left-skewed distributions in veterinary medicine.[14] The mean percentage of cattle diagnosed and treated for bovine respiratory disease (BRD) in the United States has been estimated to be 14.4%.[15] However, **Fig. 2A** shows that the mean for BRD may not completely reflect BRD morbidity outcomes when there is a right-skewed distribution. The observed differences between mean and median estimates for both morbidity and mortality shown in **Fig. 2** indicate the right-skewed distribution for these outcomes. The long right tails of these distributions show that high morbidity and mortality occurs with some cattle lots, but these lots are rare in frequency. Even although high morbidity and mortality lots occur relatively infrequently, they can have large potential impacts and therefore must be considered. Although it is tempting to manage to affect the mean, understanding the full distribution of health outcomes may enable more appropriate monitoring of outcomes and evaluation of health and economic risk management decisions.

Knowledge of the full underlying distributions of health outcomes also may allow the feedlot practitioner to better understand and manage expectations for health in feedlot populations. Based on the distribution of data, there should be an expectation that some cattle lots have high morbidity (eg, 50%), but these events should occur relatively infrequently (see **Fig. 2**A) and the expected frequency can be estimated from the distribution. When these rare events (in the tail of the distribution) occur more frequently than is expected, this may represent a signal indicating that the underlying distribution has changed. For example, a feedlot may have begun to purchase more high-risk calves, resulting in a greater percentage of lots with higher morbidity and mortality risks, and thus, expectations based on the distribution of historical data are no longer appropriate. On the other hand, if the cattle population has not changed and yet the frequency of high morbidity and mortality exceeds expectations based on the historical distribution, it may be a signal indicating a need to reassess the health management program(s).

An understanding of the underlying distributions of morbidity and mortality risks also enables the realization that when lots with high morbidity and mortality are observed, there is a good chance that the morbidity and mortality risks will be lower for subsequent lots of cattle if the population or system, and thus the expected outcome distributions, have not changed. In this situation, a newly instituted management change may be perceived to have improved morbidity and mortality risks, but only because of the natural tendency for morbidity and mortality to be low for most of the population (as indicated by the underlying distributions for these outcomes).

First treatment success and case fatality risks are 2 health outcomes frequently used to evaluate feedlot treatment programs. A favorable first treatment success has been suggested to be greater than 80%.[16,17] An acceptable BRD case fatality risk has been suggested to be 6% to 10%, but case fatality may be greater than 15% for high-risk calves.[17] **Fig. 2**C, D shows data with treatment success and case fatality means that are slightly less than these suggested levels; however, notice the distributions for these health outcomes. Neither distribution is normally distributed; therefore, the means are not very informative. Further, first treatment success is just as likely to be in the 65% to 70% category as in the 80% to 85% category. For case fatality risk, the observed outcome is just as likely to be between 15% and 20% as in the 5% to 10% category. Given these distributions, the observed outcomes for any cattle lot may just as likely occur anywhere in these wide ranges even if cattle and management factors do not change. The implication of these distributions is increased difficulty of sorting out a signal indicating a management change should be considered from noise or normal variation in the outcome of interest. Therefore, the expectations for a given cattle lot need to be managed based on the underlying distributions for these outcomes and not simply based on a suggested mean.

Fig. 2C, D shows the first treatment success and case fatality risk combined for all cattle in the data set. Further evaluation of the distributions for each therapeutic treatment protocol may be useful if different protocols result in outcomes at different ends of the distribution. Differential distributions of outcomes for otherwise similar cattle populations could indicate different effects of treatment protocols. However, this data analysis should be completed only in consideration of how the therapeutic protocols were applied to the population. For example, if cases received drug X only if rectal temperature was lower than 104°F, and received drug Y only in cases with rectal temperature of 104°F or higher, then, comparisons may not be appropriate, because the potential for confounding (described earlier) exists because there is an association between rectal temperature for first diagnosis of BRD and the probability of not finishing the production cycle.[18]

The distributions for morbidity, mortality, first treatment success, and case fatality risks are not normally distributed. Therefore, knowledge of the underlying distribution is more useful for interpretation, as well as for managing expectations, than consideration of just the mean or median estimates. Understanding the impacts of a skewed distribution, for example, and perhaps targeting resources toward affecting the tails of the distribution rather than the mean, may enable more effective health and economic risk management decisions.

TEMPORAL DISTRIBUTIONS: HEALTH EVENTS OVER TIME

A thorough understanding of the temporal distributions of health outcomes, or the distribution of health events over time, may be useful for evaluating the health of feedlot cattle populations.[19] Temporal disease patterns may be useful to determine potential biological differences among diseases or cattle populations and also to recognize potential economic impacts that may not be identified using cumulative (closeout) data.[20] The numbers of cases by days on feed or the cumulative risk by days on feed have been used to assess temporal distributions in feedlot data.[16,19,21] An evaluation of health events by days on feed can enable the feedlot practitioner to determine timing of disease peak or onset and identify potential areas for further investigation.

As an example, **Fig. 3** shows examples of 2 different temporal patterns of BRD morbidity with the same total cumulative BRD morbidity (30%) during the feeding period. These figures show the cumulative morbidity by days on feed or add the percent of the population becoming new cases over time. **Fig. 3A** is an example in which most of the BRD occurred early during the feeding period, and **Fig. 3B** is an example in which most of the BRD morbidity occurred later in the feeding period. The biological processes that drive these 2 different temporal patterns are most likely different between the 2 examples, but this would not be recognized by simply evaluating the closeout or total BRD cumulative incidence, which is the same in both examples (30%). Understanding the timing of disease occurrence, and the relative timing of potential risk factors, is critical for establishing potential causal factors (which must precede the disease events). This can also be evaluated by graphing the numbers of new cases for each period (eg, by days on feed); by developing epidemiologic curves.[16] An epidemiologic curve that indicates a point source epidemic may have different causal factors compared with a propagating epidemic. Determining the temporal relationships and the related potential biological processes may enhance

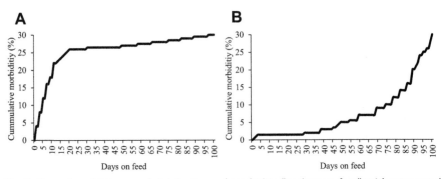

Fig. 3. Examples of 2 temporal distributions of morbidity (by days on feed) with same total cumulative morbidity risk (30%). (*A*) Most morbidity occurring early during feeding phase. (*B*) Most morbidity occurring late in feeding period.

disease detection methods, improve resource use, or enable the development of more appropriate disease control or management plans.

Knowledge of expected temporal disease patterns may also be important for considering the potential effectiveness of interventions or the potential impacts of disease on economic drivers. For example, the potential effectiveness of applying antimicrobial metaphylaxis to cattle lots when they arrive to the feedlot likely differs for different temporal patterns of BRD onset.[22] In addition, Babcock and colleagues[21] determined that there were 7 different temporal patterns of BRD within commercial feedlot cattle populations and that these patterns were associated with differences in important cattle performance indices such as average daily gain and carcass weight. It has also been shown that cattle treated with BRD later in the feeding period had decreased net returns compared with cattle treated earlier in the feeding phase.[20] These temporal analyses help show that consideration of the timing of disease occurrence is important for optimizing health interventions and evaluating impacts of disease in feedlot populations.

CONCURRENTLY ASSESSING MULTIPLE HEALTH OUTCOMES

To appropriately assess the health of feedlot cattle populations using operational data, it is often necessary to concurrently evaluate multiple outcomes. Cumulative health outcomes (ie, closeouts) are frequently formatted as percentages and are commonly used to assess the health of feedlot populations. These health outcomes often include morbidity, mortality, first treatment success, and case fatality risks. When these outcomes are used to influence health management decisions, knowledge of how they are calculated, and how they are linked with each other, is critical. To calculate these outcomes as percentages, both the numerator and denominator need to be established. The numerator is the sum of animals that met the case definition for the outcome, and the denominator is the total number of animals that were at risk for the health outcome of interest. For example, with first treatment success, the numerator is the number of calves that were treated for a disease and required no additional treatment (and finished the production cycle), and the denominator is the number of animals that were treated at least once for the disease. The same denominator may be used for the case fatality outcome measure, but the numerator is the number of those treated animals that died. Therefore, these 2 outcomes are inherently interrelated. Similarly, the numerator for a cause-specific morbidity measure, such as first treatment BRD morbidity, may be the same number as the case fatality and treatment success denominators.

These simple calculations and relationships among outcome measures are important to understand if these outcomes are being used to evaluate population health and potentially affect health management decisions. Intuitively, veterinarians tend to focus on the changing number of health events (ie, the numerators) to affect the health outcome measure. So, for example, if case fatality risk is high, the initial thought may be that the timing or efficacy of the therapeutic treatment applied is not appropriate. Both of these thoughts focus on the numerator portion of the outcome measure, reducing the number of cases that die. However, the therapy may be efficacious only if applied to animals that are truly diseased. If more animals are treated (including some that may not need treatment), the denominator for the case fatality outcome measure would increase, and the corresponding percentage value for case fatality would decrease, even when the total animals that died, or the treatment efficacy, did not change.

Table 1 provides 2 examples in which the case fatality and morbidity risks were different, but the mortality risk was the same for both examples. When case fatality

Table 1
Two example populations with different values for case fatality and morbidity for BRD, but with the same overall death loss

Example	BRD Case Fatality Risk (%)	BRD Mortality (%)	BRD Morbidity (%)	Number of Animals Died	Number of Animals Treated	Number of Animals at Risk
1	10	1	10	10	100	1000
2	5	1	20	10	200	1000

is considered in isolation, the case fatality of 5% in example 2 looks more appealing than the case fatality of 10% in example 1. However, the only reason the case fatality risk is different for these 2 examples is that more calves were treated in example 2; the number of cattle that died is the same for both examples. The additional animals treated in example 2 may not have needed treatment. Treating animals that do not need treatment can lead to an apparent improvement in treatment success and case fatality risks. However, intuitively, we know that unnecessary treatments result in increased costs without increased benefits. There are disease examples that are common in feedlot medicine, such as BRD, in which this situation can occur; more aggressive treatment programs can lead to lower case fatality and higher treatment success values, but the mortality or economic outcomes may not be improved. However, by concurrently considering multiple health outcomes (as well as performance or economic values), the assessment of the overall health of the population is more appropriate and comprehensive.

Although the examples provided in **Table 1** are hypothetical and simple situations, they do show the need to consider more than 1 health outcome to provide more accurate evaluation of feedlot health performance. The use of only 1 health outcome measure may not provide a complete picture of the health of the population, because many of the commonly used outcome measures are inherently linked (eg, through their numerators and denominators). The different outcome measures must be assessed concurrently. Percentages may be calculated from very small numbers; for example, a case fatality of 50% may seem high, but if only 1 animal died of 2 total cases, there would likely be little concern with the case fatality outcome. A systematic approach to evaluating multiple health outcomes can provide a more thorough understanding of feedlot cattle health and the importance of health management factors.

SUMMARY

Feedlot operational data may be used to develop appropriate and relevant conclusions if the data are analyzed appropriately and inferences restricted based on the limitations of the data. The operational data may be a useful resource, but the feedlot practitioner needs to be aware of how to use the data to make appropriate conclusions. Issues of data quality, potential differential errors or bias, and confounding factors must be considered to make appropriate conclusions from operational data. Knowledge of the underlying distributions of the health outcomes in the population is more useful for interpretation, as well as for managing expectations, than consideration of just the mean or median estimates. In addition, a thorough understanding of the distribution of health events over time may be useful for determining potential biological differences among disease situations or cattle populations and also for recognizing potential economic impacts that may not be identified using cumulative data. The end user of feedlot operational data may need to concurrently consider more than 1 health outcome to provide an accurate population health assessment, particularly when many of the commonly used health outcome measures are inherently linked with each other. Many potential benefits can be realized through a systematic and scientific approach to using operational data for monitoring feedlot cattle health and making valid comparisons among cattle populations.

REFERENCES

1. Lawlor DA, Smith GD, Bruckdorfer KR, et al. Those confounded vitamins: what can we learn from the differences between observational versus randomised trial evidence? Lancet 2004;363(9422):1724–7.
2. McAfee A, Brynjolfsson E. Big data: the management revolution. Harv Bus Rev 2012;90(10):60–6, 68, 128.
3. Koppel R, Metlay JP, Cohen A, et al. Role of computerized physician order entry systems in facilitating medication errors. JAMA 2005;293(10):1197–203.
4. Shelby-James TM, Abernethy AP, McAlindon A, et al. Handheld computers for data entry: high tech has its problems too. Trials 2007;8:5.
5. Day S, Fayers P, Harvey D. Double data entry: what value, what price? Control Clin Trials 1998;19(1):15–24.
6. Barchard KA, Pace LA. Preventing human error: the impact of data entry methods on data accuracy and statistical results. Comput Hum Behav 2011;27(5):1834–9.
7. White BJ. Bovine respiratory disease complex: epidemiologic methods to improve evidence-based disease management. Paper presented at: Academy of Veterinary Consultants. Colorado Springs, CO, August 2009.
8. Hogan WR, Wagner MM. Accuracy of data in computer-based patient records. J Am Med Inform Assoc 1997;4(5):342–55.
9. Hoaglin DC, Velleman PF. A critical look at some analyses of major-league baseball salaries. Am Stat 1995;49(3):277–85.
10. Dohoo I, Martin W, Stryhm H. Veterinary epidemiologic research. Charlottetown (Canada): AVC Inc; 2009.
11. Smith RA, Stokka GL, Radostits O, et al. Health and production management in beef feedlots. In: Radostits O, editor. Herd health: food animal production medicine. 3rd edition. Philadelphia: WB Saunders Company; 2001. p. 592–5.
12. Wileman BW, Thomson DU, Reinhardt CD, et al. Analysis of modern technologies commonly used in beef cattle production: conventional beef production versus nonconventional production using meta-analysis. J Anim Sci 2009;87(10):3418–26.
13. Babcock AH, Cernicchiaro N, White BJ, et al. A multivariable assessment quantifying effects of cohort-level factors associated with combined mortality and culling risk in cohorts of US commercial feedlot cattle. Prev Vet Med 2013;108(1):38–46.
14. Shott S. Detecting statistical errors in veterinary research. J Am Vet Med Assoc 2011;238(3):305–8.
15. US Department of Agriculture, Animal and Plant Health Inspection Service. Treatment of respiratory disease in U.S. feedlots. 2001.
16. Corbin MJ, Griffin D. Assessing performance of feedlot operations using epidemiology. Vet Clin North Am Food Anim Pract 2006;22(1):35–51.
17. Edwards TA. Control methods for bovine respiratory disease for feedlot cattle. Vet Clin North Am Food Anim Pract 2010;26(2):273–84.
18. Theurer ME, White BJ, Larson RL, et al. Relationship between rectal temperature at first treatment for bovine respiratory disease complex in feedlot calves and the probability of not finishing the production cycle. J Am Vet Med Assoc 2014; 245(11):1279–85.

19. Booker CW, Loneragan GH, Guichon PT, et al. Practical application of epidemiology in veterinary herd health/production medicine. Paper presented at: American Association of Bovine Practitioners. Fort Worth, TX, September 23–25, 2004.
20. Babcock AH, White BJ, Dritz SS, et al. Feedlot health and performance effects associated with the timing of respiratory disease treatment. J Anim Sci 2009; 87(1):314–27.
21. Babcock AH, Renter DG, White BJ, et al. Temporal distributions of respiratory disease events within cohorts of feedlot cattle and associations with cattle health and performance indices. Prev Vet Med 2010;97(3–4):198–219.
22. Nickell JS, White BJ. Metaphylactic antimicrobial therapy for bovine respiratory disease in stocker and feedlot cattle. Vet Clin North Am Food Anim Pract 2010; 26(2):285–301.

Index

Note: Page numbers of article titles are in **boldface** type.

A

Acclimation
    continued benefits of, 331–332
    defined, 323–324
    process of, 325–331
    purpose of, 323–325
Acute interstitial pneumonia (AIP)
    in feedlot cattle, **381–389**
        causes of, 385–386
        clinical outcomes of, 387
        defined, 381–382
        described, 381–383
        epidemiology of, 384–385
        introduction, 381–386
        pathology of, 383–384
        prevention of, 386–387
        risk factors for, 384–385
        treatment of, 386
Acute phase proteins
    in BRD diagnosis, 355
AIP. See Acute interstitial pneumonia (AIP)
Amputation
    digit
        in feedlot calves, 426–428
    tongue
        in feedlot calves, 415–416
Ankylosis of distal interphalangeal joint (DIP)
    in feedlot calves, 428–430
        plantar approach to, 428–430
        through hoof wall, 430
Antimicrobial agents
    single-injection
        in clinical evaluation of posttreatment intervals for BRD
            in calves, 447–450
Antimicrobial metaphylaxis
    in BRD control in high-risk cattle, **341–350** (See also Bovine respiratory
        disease (BRD), in high-risk cattle)
Arrival cattle management
    at feedlots, **323–340**
Automated behavior monitoring
    in early disease detection of BRD, 357–359

Vet Clin Food Anim 31 (2015) 509–519
http://dx.doi.org/10.1016/S0749-0720(15)00061-4
0749-0720/15/$ – see front matter © 2015 Elsevier Inc. All rights reserved.

vetfood.theclinics.com

Automated temperature measurements
   in early disease detection of BRD, 359

B

Bioassay for pregnancy
   feedlot
      accuracy of, 486
Biomarkers
   in BRD diagnosis, 360
Bovine respiratory disease (BRD)
   in calves
      treatment of, **441–453**
         discussion, 450–451
         duration of, 442–447
         enrofloxacin in, 447
         florfenicol in, 446–447
         introduction, 441–442
         oxytetracycline in, 446
         single-injection antimicrobials in
            clinical evaluation of posttreatment intervals for,
               447–450
      described, 351–352
      diagnosis of, **351–365**
         confirmatory diagnostics in, 354–357 (*See also* Confirmatory
            diagnostics, in BRD diagnosis)
         early detection in, 357–359
         low and wide-ranging accuracy in, 485–486
         prognostic tests in, 360–361
         systematic review of, **351–365**
            criteria for considering studies in, 352–353
            definitions for search in, 352
            implications of, 361–362
            limitations of, 361–362
            methods in, 352–353
            results and discussion in, 353–361
            search strategy in, 353
            selection of studies in, 353
   in high-risk cattle
      control of
         antimicrobial metaphylaxis in, **341–350**
            factors influencing decision to use, 343–344
            importance of, 342–343
            introduction, 341–342
            management benefits of, 345–347
            types of, 345
         preconditioning programs in, 344–345
   morbidity and mortality related to, 341
   prevalence of, 351–352
Bovine respiratory disease complex (BRDC)
   BVDv and, 368

Bovine respiratory disease (BRD) pathogens
    detection of
        in BRD diagnosis, 355–356
Bovine viral diarrhea virus (BVDv)
    BRDC and, 368
    described, 367–368
    reservoir for
        persistently infected cattle as, 368–371
    strains of
        considerations for, 371–372
Bovine viral diarrhea virus (BVDv)–associated disease
    diseases associated with, 372
    in feedlot cattle, **367–380**
        management of
            removal of persistently infected cattle in, 374–375
            testing in, 374–375
            vaccination in, 372–374
    immunosuppression associated with, 368
Bovine viral diarrhea virus (BVDv) species
    considerations for, 371–372
BRD. See Bovine respiratory disease (BRD)
BRDC. See Bovine respiratory disease complex (BRDC)
BVDv. See Bovine viral diarrhea virus (BVDv)

C

Calf(ves)
    feedlot (See Feedlot calves)
Casting
    in fracture management in feedlot calves, 432
Castration
    of feedlot calves, 408–411
Cattle
    feedlot (See Feedlot cattle)
Causal reasoning
    in investigation of outbreaks of disease or impaired productivity in
        feedlot cattle, 392–393
Ceftiofur crystalline free acid
    in clinical evaluation of posttreatment intervals for BRD in calves,
        447–448
Cesarean section
    midline
        affecting feedlot calves, 420–422
Closed fractures
    in feedlot calves
        management of, 433–434
Confirmatory diagnostics
    in BRD diagnosis, 354–357
        acute phase proteins, 355
        BRD pathogens detection, 355–356
        direct measurement of pulmonary changes, 357

Confirmatory (*continued*)
    stress-related hormones, 356–357
    WBC, 354–355
Confounding
  identifying and controlling
    in feedlot operational data, 499–501

D

Dehorning
  of feedlot calves, 411–412
Diagnostic testing strategies
  feedlot, **483–493**
    in determining positive and negative predictive values,
      486–488
    examples of, 485–486
    highly accurate, 486
    introduction, 484
    low and wide-ranging diagnostic accuracy among, 485–486
    misclassifications of
      economic consequences of, 488–490
    optimization of
      decision matrix for, 490
    retesting positive or negative animals from initial test, 490–491
    sensitivity and specificity, 484–485
Digit amputation
  in feedlot calves, 426–428
DIP. *See* Distal interphalangeal joint (DIP)
Distal interphalangeal joint (DIP)
  ankylosis of
    in feedlot calves, 428–430

E

Enrofloxacin
  for BRD in calves
    duration of, 447
  in clinical evaluation of posttreatment intervals for BRD in calves,
    449–450
Enucleation
  in feedlot calves, 412–413
Euthanasia
  feedlot, **465–471**
    captive bolt and gunshot considerations in, 467
    conditions warranting, 466
    considerations related to, 466–467
    gun in, 468–469
    intent of, 466–467
    safety of, 466–467
    secondary technique in ensuring death, 470–471
    sedative/tranquilizer use in, 467
    target aiming in, 469–470

External skeletal fixation
    in fracture management in feedlot calves, 433

F

Feeder cattle
    price discovery of, 344–345
Feedlot(s)
    arrival cattle management at, **323–340**
    diagnostic testing strategies in, **483–493** (*See also* Diagnostic testing
        strategies, feedlot)
Feedlot calves
    BVD in
        treatment of, **441–453** (*See also* Bovine respiratory disease
            (BRD), in calves, treatment of)
    common disorders of
        therapeutic options and/or surgical management of,
            407–424 (*See also specific procedures*)
            castration, 408–411
            dehorning, 411–412
            enucleation, 412–413
            introduction, 407–408
            midline cesarean section, 420–422
            perineal urethrostomy, 416–419
            rumenostomy, 419–420
            rumenotomy, 419–420
            tongue amputation, 415–416
            tracheostomy, 413–415
    orthopedic and musculoskeletal disorders of
        surgical management of, **425–439**
            ankylosis of DIP, 428–430
            digit amputation, 426–428
            for fractures, 430–435 (*See also* Fracture(s), in feedlot
                calves, management of)
            for pedal osteitis, 430
            for tendon disorders, 435–437
    pain management in, 425–426
Feedlot cattle. *See also* Feedlot calves
    AIP in, **381–389** (*See also* Acute interstitial pneumonia (AIP), in
        feedlot cattle)
    BVDv–associated disease in, **367–380** (*See also* Bovine viral
        diarrhea virus (BVDv)–associated disease, in feedlot cattle)
    disease or impaired productivity in
        investigation of outbreaks of, **391–406**
            causal reasoning in, 392–393
            challenges related to, 401–402
            communication of results of, 404
            describing outbreaks in, 395–399
            drawing conclusions from, 399–404
            finding system solution in, 403–404
            future considerations related to, 404

Feedlot (*continued*)
        important concepts related to, 392–394
        introduction, 391–392
        level of action in, 393–394
        measures of association in, 400
        measures of impact in, 402–403
        process of, 394–399
        reasons for, 394
        significance testing in, 401
        steps in, 394–395
   persistently infected
     as reservoir for BVDv, 368–371
Feedlot euthanasia, **465–471**. *See also* Euthanasia, feedlot
Feedlot necropsy, **471–481**. *See also* Necropsy, feedlot
Feedlot operational data
   in making valid conclusions for improving health management,
      495–508
      concurrently assessing multiple health outcomes in, 505–506
      distributions of population health outcomes in, 501–504
      identifying and controlling confounding in, 499–501
      introduction, 495–496
      making appropriate comparisons in, 499–501
      potential for differential errors in, 498–499
      quantity and quality of data in, 496–498
      temporal distributions in, 504–505
Feedlot processing
   arrival cattle management and, **323–340**
   described, 332–337
Feedlot records
   BRD diagnosis based on, 360–361
Feedyard hospitals
   management of, **455–463**
     animal inventory–related, 461
     feed and hay provision in, 462
     husbandry items–related, 462–463
     introduction, 455
     pen types, 455–456
     posttreatment intervals, 460
     sorting cattle in hospital, 460
     system types, 456–459
     tank and pen cleaning in, 461
     withhold times–related, 461
Florfenicol
   for BRD in calves
     duration of, 446–447
Fracture(s)
   in feedlot calves
     management of, 430–435
       casting in, 432
       closed *vs.* open fractures, 433–434
       complications of, 434–435

humerus fractures, 434
metacarpus and metatarsus III/IV fractures, 434
radius and ulna fractures, 434
splinting in, 431
Thomas splint and cast combination in, 432–433
tibia fractures, 434
transfixation pinning and casting and external skeletal
    fixation in, 433

H

Health management
  improving
    feedlot operational data in making valid conclusions for,
      495–508 (*See also* Feedlot operational data, in making valid
      conclusions for improving health management)
High-risk cattle
  BRD in
    control of
      antimicrobial metaphylaxis in, **341–350** (*See also* Bovine
        respiratory disease (BRD), in high-risk cattle)
Hoof wall
  ankylosis of DIP through
    in feedlot calves, 430
Hormone(s)
  stress-related
    in BRD diagnosis, 356–357
Hospital(s)
  feedyard (*See* Feedyard hospitals)
Hospital feed and hay provision
  in feedyard hospital management, 462
Humerus fractures
  in feedlot calves
    management of, 434

L

Laceration(s)
  tendon
    in feedlot calves
      management of, 436
Level of action
  in investigation of outbreaks of disease or impaired productivity in
    feedlot cattle, 393–394
Lung lesions
  direct indicators of
    in BRD diagnosis, 360

M

Measures of association
  in investigation of outbreaks of disease or impaired productivity in
    feedlot cattle, 400

Metacarpus III/IV fractures
   in feedlot calves
      management of, 434
Metatarsus III/IV fractures
   in feedlot calves
      management of, 434
Midline cesarean section
   affecting feedlot calves, 420–422
Musculoskeletal disorders
   of feedlot calves
      surgical management of, **425–439** (*See also* Feedlot calves,
         orthopedic and musculoskeletal disorders of)

N

Necropsy
   feedlot, **471–481**
      described, 471–473
      recording observations in, 479–481
      safety of, 473
      sharp knives in, 473–474
      technique, 473–479
      tools in, 473

O

Open fractures
   in feedlot calves
      management of, 433–434
Orthopedic disorders
   of feedlot calves
      surgical management of, **425–439** (*See also* Feedlot calves,
         orthopedic and musculoskeletal disorders of)
Osteitis
   pedal
      in feedlot calves
         surgical management of, 430
Oxytetracycline
   for BRD in calves
      duration of, 446

P

Pain management
   in feedlot calves, 425–426
Pedal osteitis
   in feedlot calves
      surgical management of, 430
Pen(s)
   feedyard hospital
      cleaning of, 461
      types of, 455–456

Perineal urethrostomy
    in feedlot calves, 416–419
Pneumonia(s)
    acute interstitial
        in feedlot cattle, **381–389** (*See also* Acute interstitial pneumonia
            (AIP), in feedlot cattle)
Preconditioning programs
    in BRD control in high-risk cattle, 344–345
Predictive values
    diagnostic testing strategies in feedlot in determining positive and
        negative, 486–488
Pregnancy
    bioassay for
        feedlot
            accuracy of, 486
Prevalence
    in determining positive and negative predictive values in feedlot,
        486–488
Protein(s)
    acute phase
        in BRD diagnosis, 355
Pulmonary changes
    in BRD diagnosis
        direct measurement of, 357

R

Radius fractures
    in feedlot calves
        management of, 434
Rumenostomy
    in feedlot calves, 419–420
Rumenotomy
    in feedlot calves, 419–420

S

Sensitivity
    in determining positive and negative predictive values in feedlot,
        486–488
    diagnostic
        feedlot, 484–485
Significance testing
    in investigation of outbreaks of disease or impaired productivity in
        feedlot cattle, 401
Spastic paresis
    in feedlot calves
        management of, 435–436
Specificity
    in determining positive and negative predictive values in feedlot,
        486–488

Specificity (*continued*)
    diagnostic
        feedlot, 484–485
Splinting
    in fracture management in feedlot calves, 431
        Thomas splint and cast combination, 432–433
Stress-related hormones
    in BRD diagnosis, 356–357

T

Temporal distributions
    in feedlot operational data, 504–505
Tendon disorders
    in feedlot calves
        management of, 435–437
            lacerations, 436
            spastic paresis, 435–436
            tendon disruption, 436–437
Tendon disruption
    in feedlot calves
        management of, 436–437
Tendon laceration
    in feedlot calves
        management of, 436
Thomas splint and cast combination
    in fracture management in feedlot calves, 432–433
Tibia fractures
    in feedlot calves
        management of, 434
Tilmicosin
    in clinical evaluation of posttreatment intervals for BRD in calves,
        448–449
Tongue amputation
    in feedlot calves, 415–416
Tracheostomy
    in feedlot calves, 413–415
Transfixation pinning and casting
    in fracture management in feedlot calves, 433
Tulathromycin
    in clinical evaluation of posttreatment intervals for BRD in
        calves, 448

U

Ulna fractures
    in feedlot calves
        management of, 434
Urethrostomy
    perineal
        in feedlot calves, 416–419

V

Vaccination
    in BVDv management in feedlot cattle, 372–374

W

WBC. *See* White blood count (WBC)
White blood count (WBC)
    in BRD diagnosis, 354–355

Moving?

Make sure your subscription moves with you!

To notify us of your new address, find your **Clinics Account Number** (located on your mailing label above your name), and contact customer service at:

Email: journalscustomerservice-usa@elsevier.com

800-654-2452 (subscribers in the U.S. & Canada)
314-447-8871 (subscribers outside of the U.S. & Canada)

Fax number: 314-447-8029

Elsevier Health Sciences Division
Subscription Customer Service
3251 Riverport Lane
Maryland Heights, MO 63043

*To ensure uninterrupted delivery of your subscription, please notify us at least 4 weeks in advance of move.

Printed and bound by CPI Group (UK) Ltd, Croydon, CR0 4YY

03/10/2024

01040490-0001